AROMAT

To Heal And Tend The Body

Robert Tisserand

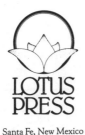

LOTUS
PRESS

Santa Fe, New Mexico

DISCLAIMER

This book is a reference work not intended to treat,
diagnose or prescribe. The information contained herein
is in no way to be considered as a substitute for consultation
with a duly licensed health-care professional.

COVER: MINA YAMASHITA GRAPHIC DESIGN
COVER PHOTOGRAPHY: MURRAE HAYNES

Library of Congress Cataloging-in-Publication Data

Tisserand, Robert.
    [Aromatherapy for everyone]
    Aromatherapy : to heal and tend the body / Robert Tisserand.
       p.   cm.
    Previously published as: Aromatherapy for everyone. 1988.
    Bibliography: p.
    Includes index.
    ISBN 0-941524-42-6 : $9.95
    1. Aromatherapy.   I. Title.
RM666.A68T565 1988
615.8'22—dc19   88-8514
                                           CIP

Published in 1988 by Lotus Press/P.O. Box 6265/Santa Fe, New Mexico 87502-6265

CONTENTS

ACKNOWLEDGEMENTS

I am indebted to a number of people for their invaluable help, in particular: Christopher Dean, Chairman of the Australian Tea-Tree Industry Association; Plaxy Kinney, Oxford Nursing Development Unit, Radcliffe Infirmary, Oxford; Arne Meander, Bio-Energetisk Institut, Rødding, Denmark; Dr Peter Nixon, Consultant Cardiologist, Charing Cross Hospital, London; Prof. Shizuo Torii, Toho University School of Medicine, Tokyo, Japan; and Dr C. Van Toller, Warwick Olfaction Research Group, University of Warwick, UK. Also to everyone who helped by providing case histories: Patricia Davis, Robert Gibson, Geraldine Howard, Susan Murdoch, Sandra Staplehurst, Christine Westwood and Valerie Worwood. And a special thanks to Sue Robinson for her many helpful suggestions with regard to text and content.

R.T.
June 1987

INTRODUCTION

> Odour is the story of language, of man's efforts to find words to express emotion and sensation. It is allied with all the senses, indissolubly with taste, with colour, sound and memory, and deeply affected by the psychological phenomenon, the power of suggestion.
>
> Edward Sagarin

During the initial long-term U S space flights the astronauts suffered from olfactory deprivation. They had nothing pleasant to smell, except for lemon-scented hand-wipes, which became highly treasured items. Soon they were not used at all for cleansing, but were saved up for sniffing sessions. Later flights purposely carried a variety of fragrant articles, and sometimes astronauts were given bottled reproductions of familiar smells from their own homes, to help prevent homesickness. Surely smell is the most evocative and yet abstract of all the senses: evocative because odours are able to conjure up emotions or memories so effectively; abstract because we have not developed a language capable of describing them. The only way we can adequately discuss them is by comparison: 'It smells like a peach' will convey something to everyone. The language of perfumery, however, is imprecise, employing words like 'green', 'floral' and 'oriental' which only describe odour types. Perhaps one reason we cannot accurately describe the smell of a peach is because odours are so evocative. We respond to them emotionally rather than intellectually. Anyone will be able to tell you right away whether they like or dislike an odour, but describing or identifying it may take more time and effort.

We use our noses much more than we probably realize.

We are surrounded by odours, pleasant or unpleasant, most of the time, and 80 per cent of what we think of as taste is in fact smell. As we eat food we taste it with our tongues, but we also 'taste' with our noses every time we exhale. Taste is a very basic sense, and all the subtle nuances of flavour are actually perceived by the nose, not the tongue. We even enjoy the smell of food without eating it. I hardly ever drink coffee, because it prevents me from sleeping, but I still find the smell of it enormously appealing and pleasurable. And of course our tastes change with time. I became a vegetarian about twenty years ago, and although I used to drool at the smell of meat cooking, I now find it distinctly unpleasant. The smell of cooking meat has not changed, but my conscious association with it has. A great many of our odour associations are personal or learned, although some of them are also instinctive. It is thought by many that infants have to learn which smells and objects should be regarded as unpleasant. Before this a baby will put *any-thing* in its mouth, even things we would regard as highly repulsive like, say, spiders or slugs. When I was about one year old I (apparently) grabbed a small bottle of French perfume, called *Crème de Zofali*, removed the glass top and promptly drank the contents. My first taste of aromatherapy.

Unlike the astronauts most of us are not deprived of pleasant odours. We find them in nature, and in many toiletries and other household items. However, we may be deprived in another sense, that of touch. In our culture, social touching is very restricted, and touching within the conventional medical system is very perfunctory. Most new-born mammals die if they are not licked by their mothers, and it has been shown that being touched is the essential factor. As adult humans we have almost as great a need to be touched. Just as pleasant odours, which most of us take for granted, are a necessary part of our well-being, so touch is a need we all share. We may compensate for lack of it by activities such as bathing or showering, changing our clothes, going to the hairdresser, crossing our legs, touching our face and so on. It is a need most of us are unaware of, or only associate with sexual activity.

Aromatherapy makes use of the two close-range senses of touch and smell. It is a pleasant therapy, but the essential oils used also have medicinal applications. Some of them, for instance, are powerful anti-microbial agents, rivalling antibiotic drugs in their effectiveness. Others have psychotherapeutic applications, relieving stresses such as depression, insomnia and pre-menstrual syndrome. Aromatherapy is one of the many ways in which the forces of nature can be made use of for the purpose of healing. At the time of writing it is not one of the best known therapies, but is probably the fastest growing in terms of popularity. Ten years ago hardly anyone had even heard of it, outside of France. Although it has a pedigree of some 5000 years, the term 'aromatherapy' was only coined in 1937, and it has only come into its own in the last twenty to thirty years, when the ancient and powerful combination of aromatic oils and massage was revived.

When I first heard the word aromatherapy I thought it sounded rather strange, and yet was intrigued. The term has been criticized as being incorrect and misleading, on the basis that it is the liquid essential oils we use, not just their aromas. In fact aromatherapy makes full use of both, and I think the word accurately conveys the concept of healing with aromatic substances. As we will see, it is a therapy of great versatility and scope, and touches on many other areas. This book aims to investigate and update the subject of aromatherapy in a way which is both interesting and understandable. While it is not a textbook for therapists, nor a do-it-yourself book for lay enthusiasts, I hope it will be keenly devoured by both. At the same time it provides a very adequate introduction for anyone curious about aromatherapy and its many facets, and includes some useful guidelines on self-treatment, or for anyone planning to go to an aromatherapist. Self-treatment is quite safe, provided that the oils are sensibly and correctly used. Self-diagnosis is not advisable, nor is self-treatment for anything moderately serious.

It has been estimated that our planet boasts in the region of 400 000 different odours. The human nose, while not as sensitive as that of many other creatures, is capable of distinguishing between each one of those odours. It would do us no harm at all to use our noses a little more consciously than we do. It is my experience that many people do not have a very developed sense of smell, because they do not use it very often. Consequently the relationships between odour and emotion, colour, taste or meaning, are not perceived. As we will see, odours do carry messages for us, and they do affect us in subtle ways, even though we may not be aware that we are smelling anything. Olfactory education is something few of us have enjoyed. We are taught how to walk, how to speak, how to play music, but the only thing most of us learn about odours is what smells bad. I believe that fragrant plants and their essential oils should form the basis of our olfactory frame of reference, rather than commercial perfumes, soaps and shampoos. Olfactory awareness and education could easily be taught in schools, and would take very little time overall. One of my two daughters, Lucy, who is now ten, has had an interest in odours since she was five. With a little guidance from Dad, she made her first perfume at six, and has an excellent nose. Olfactory awareness also improves one's taste sensitivity. As well as helping future perfumers and aromatherapists it would be of great benefit to all future cooks, professional or otherwise. Now there's a worthwhile thought.

Ultimately we are responsible for our own health. We decide what we eat, how much exercise we get, how we think, and, if we fall ill, what to do about it. Doctors and healers have always been needed, and always will be, but most of us would benefit from being a little more aware of what health involves. I do not suggest that we should all become vegetarian, jogging, teetotalling health nuts who think about nothing else. On the other hand there is more to being healthy than cutting down on smoking, red meat and white sugar, and eating 'wholemeal bread'. Massage is another area where we could help, not so much ourselves, but those close to us, and it is such a natural thing to do. Babies thrive on it, and it helps bonding with both parents. Mums and Dads should learn to massage their children. It is fun to do, promotes health in many ways and it is educational. Children also love it, and need it too. I was surprised to find that my own children, even at a young age, have the same muscular tensions as adults. Of course adults can also benefit tremendously from massage, which helps to release emotional as well as physical tensions.

Essential Oils

What exactly are essential oils, and in what sense are they 'essential'? An essential oil is what gives fragrance to a rose blossom or a sprig of rosemary. It is a liquid which is present in tiny droplets or sacs in the plant. During certain times of year, and certain times of day, there is a greater amount of essential oil in the plant, and these are the best times for harvesting and distillation. These oils are not greasy at all, in fact they are highly volatile, meaning that they readily evaporate. When heated they quickly transform from liquid to vapour, and it is the essential oil vapour which you smell when you come close to a fragrant flower or aromatic herb. However, not all flowers are fragrant, not all herbs are aromatic, so these oils are by no means essential to plant life. They are only essential in the sense that they are very concentrated. In most Germanic languages they are called 'ethereal oils' and this is really a much better term, since it evokes the subtle, almost unworldly quality which they possess.

Each essential oil has a number of different properties and uses. Lavender oil, for instance, is a gentle sedative, and may be used to relieve nervous tension, but it is also used to treat burns, headaches and many other conditions. Rosemary oil is a stimulant, and is used to aid concentration, but is also helpful in the treatment of muscular aches and influenza. Rose essential oil, sometimes known as rose *otto*, is very costly, but is enormously useful and versatile. It counteracts the damaging effects of alcohol on the liver, and helps to relieve a hangover. It also soothes feelings such as anger, envy and resentment. The fact that natural plant oils affect us emotionally is not really so very strange. Are we not universally attracted to sweet-smelling flowers like roses, hyacinths and jasmines? Do we not find their delightful fragrances to be a source of simple pleasure and contentment? Somehow these heavenly scents make us feel good inside. So the next time you start to feel irritable, angry or a bit low, indulge in the fragrance of a flower or essential oil, and experience for yourself the simple power of aromatherapy.

Some Useful Definitions

Before you read any further it will help if you understand the different meanings of these apparently similar terms:

Essential oil

A non-oily and highly fragrant essence which is extracted from a plant by distillation, and which evaporates readily. Distillation has been known since the tenth century and cannot be performed in the home.

Infused oil

A vegetable oil which has been 'infused' with the fragrance of an aromatic plant by mixing the two together and heating. The resulting oil is delicately fragrant, very greasy and does not evaporate. Infused oils have been around for at least 5000 years and can easily be made in the home.

Aromatic oil

A term which can indicate either or both of the above. Sometimes incorrectly used to describe a perfume oil.

Aromatic chemical

Essential oils consist of aromatic chemicals, put together by nature. Most essential oils have between 50 and 500 different chemical constituents. Perfumes consist of a man-made mixture of aromatic chemicals and essential oils. The chemicals used may be isolated from natural substances, but the majority are synthetic and quite a few do not occur in nature at all.

Perfume

Up until the nineteenth century all perfumes were composed of natural aromatic oils. Modern perfumes are, on average, only 20 per cent natural, the rest being synthetic aromatic chemicals. Perfumes are dilutions which today usually have an alcoholic base. A toilet water or cologne contains a lower percentage of fragrance than a perfume, and also has some water in the base.

Perfume oil

A vague term which could indicate the fragrant ingredients of a perfume, but is more commonly used to describe a perfume with a non-greasy oil base.

CHAPTER ONE

AROMATHERAPY TODAY

The cure of the part should not be attempted without treatment of the whole.

Plato, *Chronicles*

Aromatherapy may be new to you, but it is as old as the pyramids of Egypt. How such a fascinating and effective therapy managed to stay quiet and nameless for almost 5000 years still puzzles me, but the same thing seems to have happened to other healing disciplines, like reflexology. If aromatherapy has been a long time coming, it has been well worth waiting for, and all the signs are that it has, finally, arrived.

This is a holistic treatment which does not use toxic or violent remedies, and so the essential oils do not have unpleasant side-effects. It is a caring, hands-on therapy which seeks to induce relaxation, to increase energy, to reduce the effects of stress and to restore lost balance to mind, body and soul. Aromatherapy works *with* the forces of nature, not against them, and so is capable of bringing about true healing. It is not a symptom-squashing form of medicine.

Among the dozens of different treatments now being practised, aromatherapy is quite unique in one sense. It is the only one in which remedies, or medicines, are successfully combined with a body-contact therapy. In aromatherapy both aspects are equally important, whereas all other forms of healing emphasize either one or the other. It is the combination of massage and essential oils which makes it so special and so effective. Aromatherapists draw on the knowledge and benefits of both schools of thought, which sometimes gives them an unusual insight into the problems presented by a patient. It is true that some practitioners have trained in, say, both herbal medicine and acupuncture, but these are still implemented as two separate disciplines.

Just as massage can be given without using essential oils, so essential oils are sometimes employed without massage. In fact aromatherapy is practised in different ways by different types of practitioner. There are three main schools of thought, which could be defined as follows.

Holistic aromatherapy

A hands-on therapy, employing essential oils and massage for treating a wide range of disorders which may involve both mind and body. Other factors, such as nutrition and subtle energy imbalances, are usually taken into consideration too.

Medical (Clinical) aromatherapy

A prescription therapy, in which essential oils are usually given by mouth. It is commonly used for the treatment of infectious diseases by certain French doctors. Herbal preparations are often prescribed at the same time.

Aesthetic aromatherapy

The use of aromatherapy oils, often ready-blended, by beauty therapists. Treatment is given to relax, to aid in slimming or to treat skin problems such as acne and stretch marks.

One could add that self-treatment, perhaps with commercial aromatherapy products, constitutes a separate, and valid, category.

I am aware that there may be argument and also some

confusion regarding the above definitions. Many aesthetic aromatherapists would prefer to think of themselves as holistic aromatherapists, even though their aromatherapy training is often completed in a matter of three or four days. The terms 'holistic' and 'clinical' aromatherapy have already been used by others in ways which do not accord with these definitions, and clinical aromatherapists do sometimes use massage. However, I feel that some way of distinguishing the various approaches is essential. Ultimately there will have to be clear guidelines and standards of training for each one. Merely applying essential oils to the body, with no real understanding of underlying problems, causes and effects, does not constitute a form of healing. I do not wish to denigrate or discourage anyone, and aesthetic aromatherapy has a valuable role to play, but those who practise it must do so within the limits of their knowledge.

In the past aromatherapy has been described as nothing more than a form of relaxing massage, and it has been implied that there is no evidence of any real therapeutic value. Aesthetic aromatherapy has been used as the yardstick to judge the whole therapy. In fact there is abundant evidence for the healing effects of aromatherapy – anatomical, experimental, empirical, and clinical evidence – much of which is referred to in the following pages.

Aromatherapy has been described as a branch of herbal medicine (a valid description for medical aromatherapy) and as a branch of beauty therapy (valid for aesthetic aromatherapy). However, holistic aromatherapy is not a branch of anything, it is a therapy in its own right and deserves to be recognized as such. At the time of writing holistic aromatherapy is not practised by an enormous number of people, but the demand for it is growing rapidly. One obvious risk here is that there will be yet more 'quickie' courses to teach it, which will only pay lip-service to holistic principles. All the more reason why the credentials of aromatherapists should be carefully examined (see p. 145). As well as its association with herbal medicine and beauty treatments, the word aromatherapy has recently been used by elements of the fragrance industry, in connection with 'mood fragrances'. This is an unfortunate move, and is stretching the word aromatherapy beyond its natural limitations. Hopefully another name will be found to describe perfumes (mainly consisting of synthetic ingredients) which claim to evoke various moods. One group which could certainly make use of essential oils is the psychotherapists. In her *Herbal Body Book* Jeanne Rose mentions André Virél, a French psychoanalyst who worked with people unable to remember long-buried pain and traumas. He is credited with being able to bring forth such hidden memories by wafting cotton-wool balls scented with certain essential oils under patients' noses. There are many ways in which essential oils, either with or without massage, could be used to supplement the techniques of psychotherapy.

Essential oils are extremely versatile, and are used in many different contexts. They do have valid applications in beauty therapy, as medicines, as evokers of mood, and they commonly find their way into food and tobacco flavours, patent medicines, toiletries, soaps, perfumes and room fragrances. They may be used either for their taste, their fragrance, their cosmetic effect or their therapeutic power. When used therapeutically I do feel that they need a solid context, a support system, whether it be massage, psychotherapy, clinical findings or holistic analysis.

Historical Perspective

We could say that modern aromatherapy, which uses essential oils, began in Germany in the sixteenth century and that it has taken 400 years to reach its present state of development. It would also be true to say that most of this development has taken place this century. However, we must not ignore the fact that a form of aromatherapy (using infused oils) was being practised 5000 years ago, and the credit for this is probably due to an Egyptian called Imhotep, who was later deified as the god of medicine and healing. The combination of aromatic oils and massage was very common in all ancient civilizations, and formed a part of medical practice for some 4000 years. About 1000 years ago its use began to decline, and was not revived until the 1950s. In the intervening centuries essential oils were being used in many ways, including therapeutically, but invariably *not* in combination with massage. In this sense we could say that a very ancient art has been revived only very recently. So why is aromatherapy becoming so popular now?

One reason is surely that it is a relaxing, hands-on therapy. Massage is both physically and mentally relaxing, and at the same time it makes us feel emotionally nourished and cared for. Any therapy which is genuinely relaxing is going to counter the negative effect of the stresses which contribute so much to ill health today. At the same time massage is caring by its very nature. The therapeutic touch is not so very different to the loving touch of a mother for her baby, or of two lovers. It makes us feel good, and we all need to feel good; in fact it may be that aromatherapy and massage are especially effective on people who lack love in their lives, or who were rarely caressed as babies by their mothers (or fathers). An independent survey of alternative

Table 1. Percentages of patients satisfied or dissatisfied with various alternative therapies

Therapy	Satisfied	Dissatisfied
Meditation/relaxation	83	12
Massage	82	9
Psychotherapy	75	12
Osteopathy	73	14
Herbal medicine	73	18
Healing	68	16
Chiropractic	68	19
Homoeopathy	66	16
Vitamin/mineral therapy	65	12
Acupuncture	50	47
Hypnotherapy	43	50

Note: These figures are the results of an independent survey in which 2000 people were questioned. It was carried out by Research Surveys of Great Britain, a division of Europe's largest market-research organization, A G B.

therapies carried out in 1984[1] revealed that the treatments which people were most satisfied with were relaxation and massage (see Table 1).

It is important to remember, when looking at the survey results, that they are not hard success-rate figures, but rather reflect the patient's general degree of satisfaction. It may well be that the major therapies which did not score so well, notably acupuncture and homoeopathy, have a greater potential to produce more lasting health improvements in serious conditions than massage and relaxation therapy. It may also be significant that acupuncture, which some people would regard as an unpleasant treatment (although its *effects* can be very pleasant), rates very low. The two top scorers, however, are therapies which aim to make you feel good immediately.

Aromatherapy was not included in the survey but of course involves massage, with the added dimension of fragrance, so that the sense of smell, as well as the sense of touch, is prevailed upon. Aromatherapy massage is surely one of the most pleasant and relaxing therapeutic experiences. If the patient feels secure and relaxed he or she is more likely to benefit from the treatment as a whole, and of course the essential oils all possess their own healing properties, both physical and psychological. Aromatherapy can have quite a profound influence on the mind and emotions, and some very recent research is shedding light on the intricate connections between odour, brain and feeling. Essential oils are readily absorbed by the skin, and so are ideal for skin problems, and for many conditions which can be treated through the skin, such as rheumatism, muscular aches, and varicose veins. Being volatile, the oils are also well suited for inhalations to treat respiratory or sinus infections. All essential oils have anti-bacterial properties, and they do offer us a viable alternative to antibiotic drugs. In short, essential oils present us with a quite unique combination of skin permeability, volatility and fragrance, along with psychotherapeutic benefits, antisepsis and many other individual properties.

Therapy Perspective

Stress and sickness go hand in hand so often that I have devoted a separate chapter to the psychological aspects of aromatherapy (see Chapter 5). Common disorders which are stress-related, such as pre-menstrual syndrome (P M S), high blood pressure, many headaches, digestive disturbances and so on, will benefit greatly from aromatherapy. Many such problems stem from a disturbance in one or other of the everyday functions of our bodies. The normal balance of nervous tone, hormone secretion or blood pressure can be upset if too much physical or psychological pressure (*stress*) is put on our system. A certain degree of stress is a perfectly healthy thing, in fact we need it to motivate us in life. For 'stress' we could almost substitute the word 'excitement'. However, if we push things too far, or if circumstances dictate that our stress level is not being matched by adequate sleep, exercise, nutrition and emotional nourishment, then our body will start flashing a red warning light. The conventional way of dealing with this 'red light', or symptom, which might perhaps be a pain, is simply to smash the light – 'take some of these and your pain will go away'. But dealing with symptoms alone is not the answer; we need to understand what lies behind the warning light.

There is an increasing public awareness of the danger of getting hooked on tranquillizers, and their usefulness is very debatable. Aromatherapy is one of the alternative treatments for the type of problem for which tranquillizing drugs are prescribed – stresses, anxieties, depressions and so on. It is also being used to help wean people off tranquillizers, which can be very difficult (see p. 118). Aromatherapy does not remove stress, it distances us from it, and helps us to cope with it. Stress is never purely physical, or purely emotional. It is a phenomenon involving body, mind and feelings, and aromatherapy helps by balancing disturbances and strengthening weaknesses on all three levels. It is an appropriate treatment to have for what I call night-before nerves. The day before an exam, driving test, your wedding, a job interview or any similar situation is a time for aromatherapy. It is therefore especially suited to entertainers and performers, and also for sports people. Anyone who likes to work-out and keep fit will benefit from the muscle-toning, relaxing and anti-arthritic properties of essential oils in combination with massage.

The natural therapies are not based on 'magic bullets',

on natural wonder drugs. To a large extent they stimulate the body's innate healing powers, and when energies have been severely depleted the greatest care and patience is required. A body which has been ravaged for years by alcohol and tobacco, by junk food and anxiety, or by overwork and lack of rest is simply not capable of instant recovery just because the correct remedy is given. In such cases the body and mind are in an extreme state of exhaustion, and are prey to all kinds of infections, chronic diseases or behavioural breakdowns. The body needs a rest from its excesses and artificial stimulants, it needs wholesome food, fresh air, regular exercise and rest. For many people sleep is so disturbed that it does not give them the rest that they need so badly, and sleeping pills are not the answer; ultimately they only make the problem worse. Massage can be a tremendous help here, to re-educate the body in the lost art of rest and relaxation.

There is more to holistic aromatherapy than essential oils and massage; it is a healing process, in which both therapist and patient play important roles. Healing is a way of being, a way of being true to yourself and to nature, which presents a challenge for the therapist, but also a challenge for the patient. For many of us healing could almost be described as a mystical experience in which that ever elusive 'life force' plays a little game involving therapist, patient, and essential oils. It just so happens that in aromatherapy essential oils and massage are the media through which healing takes place.

Because it involves treating the patient, not just the illness, in one sense it does not matter what is wrong with you, aromatherapy can help. However, aromatherapists (apart from the French doctors) do not treat the more serious ailments such as nervous diseases (multiple sclerosis, Parkinsonism, epilepsy etc.), cancers and serious infections such as hepatitis, diphtheria, meningitis, AIDS, venereal diseases and so on. Aromatherapy is of considerable help in the area of common, stress-related and other minor disorders for which the busy general practitioner often finds it difficult to provide a solution. These include such conditions as menopausal and menstrual disorders, including PMS, moderate anxiety/depression, sleeping problems, impotence/frigidity, minor aches and pains, digestive disorders, migraines, skin problems such as acne and eczema, and minor infections such as cystitis, vaginal or throat infections and acute bronchitis. Aromatherapy can also be of great assistance in slightly more serious conditions, where the co-operation of a doctor is sometimes necessary.

Aromatherapy can help in acute diseases just as much as in chronic ones. For instance, self-treatment with inhalations can be of enormous benefit for colds, flu and acute bronchitis, although it is always best in such cases to check with your aromatherapist that you are doing the right thing. Emotional disturbances can also be alleviated, although if these are of a very serious nature it would be best to consult an expert such as a psychotherapist. (Remember that food allergies can sometimes cause mental disturbances.) Aromatherapy can help the very young, although extra care needs to be exercised when using essential oils to treat under-fives. It can also help the elderly, who often have their own particular problems. Some aromatherapists do home visits, and this is obviously helpful for those who find it physically difficult to go out. Aromatherapy can be very useful during pregnancy, although again extra care needs to be exercised, and also in post-natal care, which for some is the time when they need help the most.

Because they treat causes as well as symptoms, natural

therapies are often preventive, that is to say they nip disease in the bud. The minor problems that we have already discussed, sleep disturbances, digestive disorders and so on, could eventually lead to something much more serious. With aromatherapy we can rebalance those areas where harmony has been disturbed, such as the endocrine system, which controls the secretion of hormones, the immune system, which fights off infection, and the nervous system, which itself controls many bodily functions such as blood pressure. By utilizing skills like muscle-testing and reflexology we can detect a weakening in an organ or area of the body long before things have reached the stage of clinical, classifiable disease. The barometer is simply how you feel. If you do not feel as good as you should, pay a visit to a therapist, and, if and when you feel better, you know that something positive has happened to you, even though you may not fully understand what. Prevention really is better than cure. It is much simpler, it saves you a lot of trouble and it is cheaper.

Aromatherapy is compatible with all other natural therapies, with the possible exception of homoeopathy. However, most practitioners prefer you to stick to one therapy at a time. If, for instance, you are visiting an acupuncturist and an aromatherapist, neither is going to know how much effect their treatment is having. As things develop we may see a change in attitude, and more co-operation between different types of practitioner. With homoeopathy there is a certain incompatibility. It is thought that essential oils negate the healing powers of homoeopathic remedies, which are very subtle. Whether this applies to all essential oils or only a few is a matter of conjecture, but no doubt this will become clear in the fullness of time. For the moment the two therapies should not be combined. There are many reasons why aromatherapists and the medical profession should work more closely together, and such a move would certainly be in the best interests of the patient. Already there are isolated pockets of co-operation; let us hope that this continues to develop.

Whether essential oils are compatible with chemical drugs depends on how we interpret the word 'compatible'. As far as we know there are no dangerous combinations, so you do not run any risks by combining the two. On the other hand they do tend to work in different ways rather than harmoniously, and if you are taking any strong drugs they will probably have a dampening effect on any aroma-therapy treatment.

There is a strong case for the use of essential oils in hospitals. First, because they are both volatile and anti-septic, they are the ideal weapon against the spread of air-borne infection, a problem in many hospitals. (Essential oils were used in this way in a few French hospitals in the 1930s.) Second, aromatherapy could be useful in so many ways to nurses, health visitors and anyone who has regular, direct contact with patients, and there are signs that this is beginning to happen. At the Oxford Nursing Development Unit of the Radcliffe Infirmary in Oxford patients often receive aromatherapy massage, under the direction of nurse practitioners. In the same part of the hospital, oils of ger-anium, lavender, lemongrass and tea-tree are being tried out instead of chemical disinfectants and antiseptics. Could this be the beginning of a trend towards a more healthy medical atmosphere?

A Female Phenomenon?

At the time of writing women far outnumber men in aromatherapy, whether we look at practitioners, patients or those who use essential oils at home. In the UK this can be ascribed to the fact that aromatherapy has received most of its publicity in the women's press, and aesthetic aroma-therapy is now widely practised in beauty salons. How-ever, the situation is changing, and if we look at France, where clinical aromatherapy is well established among the medical profession, neither sex predominates. As a cosmetic treatment it naturally appeals more to women, but as a therapeutic one – well, is there any reason why women should benefit more than men?

A Dutch Government report published in 1983[2] showed that women's skin is more permeable to toxic chemicals than men's skin. This means that female skin is also more permeable to essential oils, not because they are toxic, but because they are skin-permeable. However, this only applies to undiluted oils – as soon as they are mixed in vegetable oil, which is the way they are used in aroma-therapy, the difference no longer applies. In practice we find that skin absorption capability does vary from one person to another, but has absolutely nothing to do with sex. Female skin might still absorb better when essential oils are used with water, as in compresses or baths, but if there is a difference it is only a small one.

The Dutch report also reminds us that women carry twice as much body fat as men – 20–25 per cent of total body weight as opposed to 10–15 per cent in men. This, it is concluded, would mean that fat-soluble substances (such as essential oils) would remain in the female body for longer. This seems logical, and may well give women a slight advantage as patients. However, obesity would surely be a problem, since the oils would have to penetrate through so much fatty tissue before they could reach the organs needing treatment. A study conducted in 1956[3] showed that obese people have a less acute sense of smell than those of normal weight, so obesity is certainly not a plus in aromatherapy. Treatment, especially for psychological or stress-related problems, relies on the patient smelling and inhaling the odour, as well as on skin absorption, so an acute sense of smell might enable some patients to benefit more from treatment.

A comparative study carried out in 1970[4] concluded that women have a more acute sense of smell than men, and that it is at its sharpest in the morning. Whether smell sensitivity makes any difference to emotional responsiveness is debatable, but, if it does, then women with stress-related problems might well benefit more from treatment earlier, rather than later, in the day. Curiously, women's sense of smell deteriorates as the day unfolds, but that of men remains steady, and by late afternoon is equal to that of women. Men, therefore, would benefit equally from treatment, regardless of the time of day. Age is another factor in smell sensitivity, and it has been shown that our sense of smell gradually fades as we advance in years.[5]

It is worth mentioning here that aromatherapy is an especially appropriate treatment for helping in pregnancy, and for most 'female disorders'. We have already mentioned its effectiveness in treating vaginal infections and all types of menstrual disorders, and it can also be of help in problems related to the menopause. In pregnancy aromatherapy helps to relieve many of the minor irritations, such as morning sickness and backache, and the massage part is especially useful in preparing the body of the mother-to-be for birth. Labour pains, stretch marks and post-natal depression can all be minimized with aromatherapy. Re-toning the body after birth and helping to balance out mood swings can be the most important part of all.

CHAPTER TWO

NOTHING NEW

That which has been is that which shall be; And that which is done shall be done; And there is nothing new under the sun.

Ecclesiastes 1

The story of aromatherapy begins with the most ancient civilizations, and it starts with an enigma which could help to throw a new light on the ancient history of mankind. In the Taxila Museum, Pakistan, there is an object made of terracotta which experts have judged to be 5000 years old.[1] There can be no doubt what this object was used for; it is a still, and would have been used for making aromatic waters, and perhaps essential oils from plants. The puzzling part is that distillation was only invented 1000 years ago, and in the intervening 4000 years there is no evidence that distillation was known anywhere in the world. The terracotta still, which was found alongside a number of perfume and cosmetic containers, must have belonged to the ancient Indus or Arab civilizations. Could it be that, 5000 years ago, the people of that area were much more advanced than has been thought up till now?

In his book *Secrets of the Lost Races*[2] Rene Noorbergen puts forward a fascinating hypothesis which completely upsets our concepts of ancient history. He suggests that a very advanced civilization inhabited our planet thousands of years ago, and that this was all but destroyed by a massive flood – *the* Flood referred to in the Old Testament. The Flood happened 5000 years ago, to the nearest few hundred years, and the survivors were able to retain very little of their previous technology. However, a few objects have survived which tend to support this theory.

The dynastic (civilized) period of ancient Egypt stretched over some 3000 years, during which time it went through many changes. Here, if anywhere, we should expect to find some evidence of this almost lost technology, incongruously mixed with the inevitable fall into a primitive state of living. The very existence of the pyramids poses some obvious questions which have yet to be answered. We still do not know how they were constructed; even today such a task would be almost impossible. They were built with incredible accuracy, and the planners and builders must have possessed an advanced knowledge of mathematics, architectural technique and transportation.

In the nineteenth century Auguste Mariette, a French archaeologist, found some ancient gold jewellery near the Sphinx. It had been produced either by electroplating or by some similar process. Electroplating was not invented until the nineteenth century. Ancient electric batteries, dating from 250 and 650 BC, have been found in Iraq, and a model plane was discovered in 1898, in a tomb near Saqqara, Egypt. It was reckoned to be at least 2200 years old and, since aeroplanes had not yet been invented in 1898, it was classed as a 'bird object'. In 1969 the object was rediscovered in the basement of the Cairo Museum, and recognized for what it really was. Examined by aerodynamics engineers, the 'Saqqara bird' was found to be much more than a toy plane. It was a scaled-down replica, precise in every detail, of an aerodynamically perfect aircraft. This would seem to indicate the ancient existence of the real thing, and it is thought that the model represented an aircraft used to transport large amounts of freight. Could such planes have been used for transporting blocks of stone for pyramid building?

The terracotta still is another artifact which, like the 'Saqqara bird', is a mute hint of an even greater knowledge. Who made it and why? Was it used for perfumery or aromatherapy? Were essential oils and aromatherapy being used over 5000 years ago, before the Flood? The very fact that distillation was *not* known for 4000 years after the discovery of the still supports the idea that the knowledge behind its manufacture came from an even earlier period. It was probably fashioned at a time when the knowledge of distillation was in the process of being lost, only to be rediscovered thousands of years later.

Egypt

According to the orthodox view of history, civilization began with the ancient Egyptians, some 5300 years ago. The oldest pyramid in Egypt, the Step Pyramid, was built in the third dynasty, around 3000 B C, by King Zoser, whose name means 'holy'. According to Greek tradition Zoser had an extensive knowledge of things medical, but his chief architect, a man named Imhotep, was also a physician of renown. Imhotep was the first, and remains one of the few, non-royals who are remembered from early Egypt. He designed and was responsible for building the first pyramid, and is credited with the very rapid development of architecture at the time. He has been described as an original thinker and genius, and he must have been a remarkable man: chief architect, physician to the king, astronomer, scribe (all his writings have sadly been lost), Chancellor to the King, and High Priest of Heliopolis. He was later revered as the patron of scribes, and was even deified and worshipped as the god of medicine and healing. He certainly did much to advance medical knowledge, and, since infused oils and aromatic unguents were so often used in Egyptian medicine, we could justifiably label him as the grandfather of aromatherapy. King Zoser was buried at Saqqara, the site of the Step Pyramid, and also the place where the 'bird' was found. There is also a physician's tomb, with a wall painting depicting massage, but this was not Imhotep's whose resting place has never been found. The wall painting (see Figure 1) depicts a type of pressure-point massage, with characteristic contact using the tips of fingers and thumb. It could be a type of acupressure, but seems more likely to be reflexology, which is done on the hands, as well as the feet.

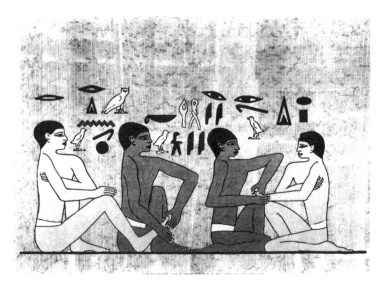

Figure 1. An Egyptian wall painting, dating from 2330 BC, from the tomb of Ankhmahor at Saqqara. The hieroglyphics read: 'Do not hurt me' (patient) and 'I shall act so you praise me' (practitioner). (Reproduced by kind permission of the International Institute of Reflexology)

One of the few surviving medical papyri is the *Papyrus Ebers*,[3] and it also provides the most valuable insight into Egyptian medicine. It is said to have been discovered in a tomb, and was published in Germany by Georg Ebers in 1875. Its date has been fixed at around 1550 BC, and much of it is thought to be a compilation of more ancient works, perhaps including some of Imhotep's writings. The papyrus is full of recipes and remedies for all kinds of ailments, and the methods of application used are not very different to those used in herbal medicine and aromatherapy today. Medicines were taken by mouth for internal diseases, external applications were used for pain, ointments for skin diseases, inhalations for respiratory problems, gargles for mouth disorders, sitz baths and douches for gynaecological problems and enemas for intestinal affections. Aromatics often feature in the various medicines, although essential oils did not appear to be known to them. Aromatic plants and gums were made into oils and ointments by infusing them. This means placing the plant in oil or fat, and leaving the mixture out in the sun for a few days. The heat transfers the fragrance of the plant to the oil or fat, along with some of its medicinal value. Aromatics were used for magical and mystical, as well as medicinal purposes, and the dividing line between these three was often indistinct.

The Egyptian healers were divided into three categories. There were the physicians, who prescribed remedies, the surgeons, who performed operations, and the sorcerers, who used magic charms or exorcisms. Many of these, especially in earlier times, were also priests. They looked for inspiration in their art to the goddess Sachmet, or the god Imhotep, and worshipped at shrines dedicated to them. It was normal to chant spells and prayers to the gods on applying a remedy. A Babylonian tablet from an earlier period bears this incantation for fever: 'Burn cypress and herbs; that the great gods may remove the evil; that the evil spirit may stand aside.'

Probably the very earliest use of aromatics was as incense. (The word perfume comes from the Latin *per fumum*, meaning 'through smoke'.) Since smoke rises to heaven, it was considered the natural vehicle to carry prayers and offerings to the abode of the gods. Altogether the Egyptians had some sixty gods and goddesses, and some of their aromatics were consecrated to various deities. Frankincense was linked with the sun, and was burned at sunrise as an offering to Ra, the sun-god, while myrrh was consecrated to the moon. Frankincense was also a popular ingredient in cosmetics, and myrrh was used in embalming. Considering their everyday use in magic, medicine and healing it is not surprising that precious gums like these two became highly valued.* The modern equivalent would possibly be the very costly oils of rose and jasmine, although they do not quite have the same mystical connotations.

One of the earliest and most celebrated aromatic formulas was a mixture of sixteen aromatics known as *kyphi*. Originally it was made as a solid incense, and was burned at sunset as an offering to Ra. It must have been very popular, as it became a common item in Egyptian homes (instead of just temples) and was later used as a liquid perfume by both the Greeks and Romans. According to C. J. Thompson⁴ kyphi was 'not only used to give an agreeable perfume to the body and clothes, but was also burned in the house to make it smell sweet, *and was employed as a*

---

* It is interesting to note that the principal ingredients of gums like frankincense and myrrh, *resin alcohols*, are very similar in chemical structure to human steroids – the male and female hormones. Whether the resin alcohols have any aphrodisiac or hormone-stimulating effect has not been proven, but it may be that there is more to man's liking for incense than religious associations.

medicine' (my italics). An explanation of its popularity can possibly be found in the words of Plutarch, a Greek historian, who said of kyphi: 'Its aromatic substances lull to sleep, allay anxieties, and brighten dreams. It is made of things that delight most in the night.'

It sounds as if kyphi, possibly the earliest recorded popular perfume, was also the original 'opium of the masses'. It certainly appears to have had soporific and narcotic properties. We cannot be certain of its exact ingredients, but most authorities agree that they include calamus,* myrrh, juniper, mastic, cinnamon, cassia, spikenard, cyperus (not cypress) henna, terebinth and perhaps frankincense and saffron. One of the sealed flasks discovered when the tomb of Tutankhamun was opened in 1922 contained an unguent which, after 3300 years, still had a perceptible odour. Analysis revealed the presence of frankincense and spikenard. Perhaps this is the only surviving bottle of the world's first perfume.

Apart from their incredible pyramids, the ancient Egyptians are probably best remembered for their mummies. Because they believed that the dead would still need their earthly bodies in the afterlife, they went to enormous lengths to preserve the body and to bury any items that might be needed along with the corpse. Many of the major organs were cut out, and the cavities were filled with cassia and myrrh. The body was drained of blood and left to dehydrate in a bath of natron. After about seventy days it was removed, given cosmetic attention and then wrapped in hundreds of metres of linen bandages impregnated with cedarwood oil and other aromatics.[5] Before burial the body

---

* If kyphi was indeed narcotic, this could be ascribed to this ingredient. Seventy-five per cent of calamus oil consists of a substance called *asarone*, which is a powerful sedative and can cause hallucinations. Calamus oil is also highly toxic and is not used in aromatherapy.

was decorated with flowers, and the ceremony ended with a prayer to the god Horus, who was requested to honour the dead person by bestowing his perfume on the body.

The ancient Egyptians became experts at the process of embalming, which has helped to highlight the antiseptic and 'flesh-preserving' properties of aromatics. Frankincense oil is one of several 'rejuvenating' essential oils employed in aromatherapy, although, paradoxically, it was never used by the Egyptians for embalming. They believed that cedarwood was imperishable, and that it would preserve anything enclosed with it or infused by its oil. It was in great demand for making temple doors and artifacts, for shipbuilding (to preserve the lives of sailors) and for coffins. The oil was used in embalming, and was smeared over papyrus leaves to protect them from insects.[6] The modern equivalent of this particular species of cedarwood is used for its antiseptic properties in respiratory and urinary infections, and has been used to treat tuberculosis and eczema.

The Egyptians were very fond of bathing, and also of massage, which usually followed a bath. After her bath the well-to-do Egyptian lady would lie naked while slave girls massaged her with fragrant oils. This, the earliest form of aromatherapy massage, served to relax, to perfume the body and to condition the skin. Cedarwood oil was frequently used, but they had other favourites too, including oils made from lilies, henna and cinnamon. 'Egyptian perfume' later became a very fashionable item in Greece, much as 'French perfume' has been for many years in modern Europe.

Greece and Rome

The ancient Greeks further sophisticated the use of aromatic oils and ointments, and employed them cosmetically
and medicinally as well as for their fragrance. Marestheus,
a physician, was possibly the first to recognize that aromatic
flowers have either stimulating or sedative properties. He
mentions *rose* and *hyacinth* as being refreshing, invigorating
a tired mind, and *lily* and *narcissus* as soporific, causing one
to feel languid. Narcissus oil is occasionally used today in
aromatherapy for its sedative action. The Greeks believed
that a perfume made from vine leaves would promote
mental alertness, while a violet perfume would often have
the opposite effect, and could send one off to sleep.
Theophrastus commented on the therapeutic nature of
perfumes, saying: 'It is to be expected that perfumes should
have medicinal properties in view of the virtues of their
spices. The effect of plasters and of what some call poultices
prove these virtues, since they disperse tumours and
abscesses and produce a distinct effect on the body and
also its interior parts.' Here he has observed one of the
fundamentals of holistic aromatherapy, the fact that
oils applied *externally* can affect the *internal* organs and
tissues.

Pedacius Dioscorides, of Anazarba in Cicilia, wrote a
magnificent treatise on herbal medicine during the first
century AD.[7] His book remained a standard medical reference work in Western medicine for over 1000 years after
his death, and much of our present knowledge of medicinal
herbs originates from Dioscorides. His book has five sec-
tions, one of which deals with aromatics, and contains a
wealth of aromatherapeutic information, including both
single and compound aromatics. Many of the remedies he
discusses are still used today in aromatherapy, for instance:

Myrrh 'Doth strengthen the teeth and ye gummes' and is 'soporiferous'.

Juniper is described as 'diureticall'.

Marjoram is described as 'soporific'.

Cypress 'The flux of the belly (diarrhoea). It doth also stanch the bloud.'

Costus 'Provokes venerie' (aphrodisiac)

As any aromatherapist will confirm, marjoram is one of the most potent sedatives, juniper is one of the best diuretics, and the astringent properties of cypress make it very useful in cases of diarrhoea. Costus, while a very reliable aphrodisiac, is now wisely avoided, since it can cause violent allergic skin reactions.

Many of the compound aromatic formulas either became or already were very popular items, just as kyphi had been in Egypt. *Susinon,* made from lilies with myrrh, calamus and cardamom, was used as a diuretic and for vaginal inflammations. *Amarakinon* contained many ingredients including cinnamon, myrrh, spikenard and costus. It was used to stimulate menstruation and to treat haemorrhoids, and it was reckoned to 'assuage and subdue ye winde'. *Nardinon muron,* or spikenard ointment, also included myrrh, costus and cardamom. It was employed for coughs, colds and 'ye losse of the voyce'. Aromatherapy may have started in Egypt, but the Greeks developed it considerably. Dioscorides also mentions kyphi: 'Cyphi is the composition of a perfume, wellcomme to ye Gods: the Priests in Egypt doe use it abundantly. It is mixt also with Antidots, and is given to the Asthmaticall in drinkes.' Since it was soporific kyphi would help to calm panic attacks, and its many antispasmodic ingredients could feasibly relieve the bronchial spasm of an asthma attack.

Dioscorides ascribes many properties to a particular

species of juniper, *Juniperus phoenicea*. It was said to kill intestinal worms, lice and 'gnittes'. It also kills worms in the ears, 'and doth quiet their noyse and hissings'. And perhaps most interesting of all, 'Being anointed about the Genitall before Conjunction it doth cause sterilitie.' So this phoenician juniper oil was used as a spermicide 2000 years ago.*

Aromatics were in great demand in ancient Greece and Rome. One Greek writer stated that: 'The best recipe for health is to apply sweet scents to the brain.' Myrrh was chewed 'for the stincking of the breath', and *kankamon*, an aromatic wood, was reported 'to have ye power of making fatt bodies leane'. In Rome the *hetairi*, or prostitutes, used scent liberally, as did many Roman Emperors. Caligula spent enormous sums on scented ointments, and was a great believer in the efficacy of aromatic baths to restore a body jaded by sexual excesses. The Greeks and Romans also believed that aromatics could temper the narcotic effects of alcohol and help to prevent hangover. This led to the use of myrrh, violets or roses in flavouring wine, and roses and rose dishes were always in abundance at the famous feasts and orgies.†

Hippocrates lived some 500 years before Dioscorides, about 2500 years ago. In his *Aphorisms*[8] we find a rare reference to aromatics: 'Aromatic baths are useful in the treatment of female disorders.' He was also keen on massage: 'The physician must be experienced in many things, but assuredly in rubbing ... For rubbing can bind a joint that is too loose, and loosen a joint that is too rigid.' Hippocrates is often referred to as the father of medicine, but it

* However, do not try using ordinary juniper oil as a spermicide; it will not work, and might result in an unpleasant irritation.
† We now know that rose oil has a specific healing effect on the liver, and it may indeed be of use in preventing or relieving hangover.

would be much more fitting to dub him the father of holistic medicine. Some 300 years after him lived a Greek physician who was perhaps closer to our concept of an aromatherapist than either Hippocrates or Dioscorides. Asclepiades was a great believer in massage. He has even been credited with originating it, although of course it was being used long before his time. He practised in both Greece and Rome, was a close friend of Cicero, and had some unusual views about healing. He believed in curing his patients with as little discomfort as possible, and was against the excessive use of purgatives and emetics, so much an integral part of medicine at that time. Instead he advocated the use of massage, music and perfume as soothing and healing agents, and he also believed that bathing and wine had curative properties.

China

It is possible that the ancient civilizations of India and China were practising some form of aromatherapy at the same period as the Egyptians. Evidence of sophisticated settlements dating back to around 3000 B C have been found in several areas of the Middle East and Far East. It has been recorded that 5000 years ago the Chinese living along the banks of the Yellow River were using calamus roots and mugwort leaves as hygiene aids. They also burned aromatic woods and herbs as incense to show reverence to God and to their forebears. We know that aromatic herbs and massage were being made use of in China at this early period, and so we could speculate that they learned to make infused oils, and so combined the two, like the Egyptians.

According to Eastern tradition the art of healing in China was founded by three legendary Emperors: Huang Ti, Shen

Nung and Fu Hsi. The oldest surviving medical text in China is Shen Nung's *Herbal*, which is dated at around 2700 BC. This book is comparable in stature to Dioscorides' *Opus Magnus*, and contains information on 365 plants, including ginseng (ginseng does contain an interesting essential oil, but it is not commercially extracted). Another of the three Emperors also penned a significant work, the *Huang Ti Nei Ching Su Wen*. This has been translated into English, and is entitled *The Yellow Emperor's Classic of Internal Medicine*.[9] The original has been dated to around 2650 BC and contains several references to massage, for example: 'When the body is frequently startled and frightened, the circulation in the arteries and the veins ceases, and disease arises from numbness and the lack of sensation. In order to cure this, one uses massage, and medicines prepared from the lees of wine.' * This almost sounds like a description of a state of stress, although the reference to *numbness* is significant, since elsewhere the author refers to massage as the treatment of choice for 'complete paralysis and chills and fever'. Massage is a traditional and logical treatment for numbness or paralysis.

Reading Huang Ti's book is a little bit like reading the Book of Revelations. It sounds incredibly wise and true and semi-mystical, but no one could pretend that they completely understand it. It does form much of the basis for acupuncture treatment, although the instruction it contains is as much philosophical as practical. However, the book is strong evidence of an even older wisdom. A system as complex as acupuncture could only be developed by a very sophisticated and enlightened civilization. There is no doubt that acupuncture works, and the existence of the meridians and acupuncture points has now been proved.

---

* There is an essential oil made from the lees of wine; it is known as *cognac oil*.

This book, therefore, is further evidence that Noorbergen's theory is correct, and that there did exist an advanced civilization which was wiped out some 5000 years ago, only traces of it surviving.

India

The oldest form of Indian medicine is known as *ayurvedic*, meaning 'knowledge of longevity'. Nobody can be sure exactly how old it is, but it has been practised for at least 3000 years, and is still widely practised in India today. One of the principal aspects of ayurveda is aromatic massage. Sometimes essential oils are used, especially oil of sandalwood which is readily available and is mentioned in the earliest ayurvedic texts. Much more common is the use of infused oils made from indigenous plants. It is doubtful whether most ayurvedic practitioners have even heard of aromatherapy, and yet that is what they are using, in their own way. Different aromatic herbs and woods are selected to make up the infused oils according to the type of problem to be treated, and the oil is then massaged, usually over the whole body, by the massage therapists. Different massage techniques are used, but mostly a fairly vigorous type of soft-tissue massage is performed. Many cures are claimed for this type of treatment on people who could not be helped by conventional medicine. Pressure-point massage is still used in India to some extent, but in traditional ayurvedic therapy it was given greater importance, and a common practice called *marma* involved massaging more than 100 points on the skin.

The Middle East

The invention of distillation is credited to the Persians, in particular to a physician and alchemist called Ibn Sina, known in the West as Avicenna (AD 980–1037).[10] Perfumed waters had been in use for many centuries, and in the ninth century these were produced by a primitive type of distillation. Rose water was by far the most popular, and the Persians exported it to China, India and Europe. It was certainly used for medicinal purposes, as well as to flavour all kinds of culinary delicacies and for finger-dipping or sprinkling over guests at dinner. Today rose water is as much in demand as ever in the Middle East, and is used for much the same purposes.

Distillation was not completely invented by one person, and took perhaps 100 years to develop. The same process results in both an aromatic water and an essential oil, and Avicenna sophisticated and refined the process and first made it possible to extract the pure essential oil. It is said that his first successful distillations were made from *Rosa centifolia*. This new development led to an even greater popularity for rose water and for the 'perfumes of Araby'. The Arabs made great advances in chemistry at around this time, and also discovered how to make alcohol. With both alcohol and essential oils the production of perfumes without a heavy, oily base became possible for the first time. As well as roses, violets, lilies, narcissi and lotus flowers were used in this new perfumery. In the thirteenth century Damascus became one of the main centres of rose-water production using a different type of rose, to which the city gave its name, the damask rose.

Interest in the therapeutic applications of essential oils was relatively small, but aromatherapy as we know it today was quietly being born. Avicenna was, like Hippocrates and Dioscorides, one of the great physicians of ancient times. He was later dubbed the 'Prince of Physicians' and it has been said that he had a mind like Goethe's and the genius of Leonardo da Vinci. During his wandering life he became the principal court physician and wrote almost 100 books. His greatest work was *Al Q'anun*, or the *Canon of Medicine*, which remained a standard reference work for some 500 years after his death. The book is reminiscent of the Yellow Emperor's work and much of it is philosophical, mystical and timeless in its wisdom. In the 'Materia Medica' section he refers to many essential oils, including cinnamon, coriander, clove, aniseed, dill, camomile, juniper and peppermint.

Avicenna was not a great believer in massage, but he did recommend it for a few particular conditions: to prepare the body for exercise, to treat lassitude after exercise, to increase or decrease body weight (different types of massage), and to give tone to the body, and for infants and the very old. As a sequel to exercise, he comments: 'Restorative friction. This produces repose. Its object is to disperse the effete matter formed in the muscles and not expelled by the exercise. It causes them to disperse and so removes fatigue. Such friction is soft and gentle and is best done with oil or perfumed ointments.'[11] We know that massage does, in fact, help to disperse certain chemicals like lactic acid, which build up in muscle tissue during exercise. He also recommended the use of *calefacient* (warming) medicines along with massage. These include essential oils of dill, camomile and willow. For reducing obesity he prescribed a regimen based on baths, dieting and massage with an infused oil based on wild cucumber, gentian, all-heal root, birthwort root and centaury. Alternatively an ointment was used based on the essential oil of dill.

Europe

There can be no doubt that the inhabitants of Europe were using herbs medicinally from the earliest times. Due to the lack of surviving records we do not know whether infused oils were known in Europe before the invasion of the Romans in the first century AD. With them the Romans would also have brought the knowledge of the healing properties of these oils; knowledge handed down and refined since the time of Dioscorides. However, the fall of the Roman Empire signalled a general decline in the level of civilization in Europe, and most of the Romans' 'aroma-therapeutic knowledge' was lost for a time. The Middle Ages, or Dark Ages, was a time when the Saxons of England were haunted by Danish invasions, and by tales of evil powers, trolls, and phantoms. In her book *The Old English Herbals* Eleanor Sinclair Rohde captures the mood perfectly: 'A supernatural terror brooded over the trackless heaths, the dark mere pools were inhabited by water elves. In the wreathing mists and driving storms of snow and hail they saw the uncouth moor gangers ... the stalking fiends of the lonely places.'[12] The Saxons were basically Christians, but were still swayed by superstitions and beliefs going back to Celtic times and beyond.

The earliest Saxon book dealing with herbs is the *Leech Book of Bald*, dating from about 900 AD. Of course all books were still written by hand and in Latin, and were only read by very few. In the twelfth and thirteenth centuries Latin transcripts of Dioscorides and other early writers began to be copied and read once more. In the fourteenth century came the small beginnings of a revival. Books written in semi-Chaucerian English, and mentioning the occasional infused oil, appeared. Some time during the fifteenth century what was probably the first comprehensive work on infused oils was written. Its author is unknown, and it is simply titled *An Herbal*. It begins: 'Here begynnyth the makynge of oyles of divrse herbys for dyvrse infirmytees and first we shall describe the makyng of oyle laurel.'* Infused oil of ivy berries is recommended for gout, oil of juniper for fever and aching kidneys, and oil of henbane for promoting sleep. Many of the oils described in this book, and in others, were for arthritis, gout, muscular aches, infected wounds and sores, and to aid in both conception and birth. The general impression one gets from these works is that their authors were far less enlightened than the celebrated Greek and Persian physicians, for whom Europeans now held a great respect.

The Sixteenth Century

The turn of the sixteenth century saw the first printed books, which gave rise to a new era for progress and the spread of knowledge. During this century Queen Elizabeth I came to the throne in England, Sir Francis Drake defeated the Spanish Armada, the first plague hit Europe and nobody washed. They wore perfume instead. Not only were bodies hardly ever bathed, but the fancy, fashionable puffed-out clothes were rarely cleaned. Consequently perfumes were in great demand. These often took the form of powders, although fragrant waters and alcoholic perfumes were also splashed liberally around. 'Strewing herbs' were in common use. These were strewn on the ground to be walked on, both for their disinfectant and aromatic qualities. Lavender, camomile, basil, melissa and thyme were all commonly strewn and trodden, both indoors and out. Lawns grown with camomile were also

* This, and other oils from the book are detailed in *The Art of Aromatherapy*.[13]

popular; 'though the camomile, the more it is trodden on, the faster it grows, yet youth, the more it is wasted, the sooner it wears' (Shakespeare, *King Henry the Fourth, Part I*, Act 2, Sc. iv).

This century also saw a great step forward for aromatherapy, which took place in Germany. This was the first real progress since the time of Avicenna, and the central figure was a man called Hieronymus Braunschweig, sometimes known as Jerome of Brunswick, but I like to refer to him as H.B. He was a physician who wrote several books on distillation, and also a few on surgery. His first work appeared in 1519, and his last great work, the *New Vollkomen Distillierbuch* was published in 1597.[14] It includes reference to twenty-five essential oils including rosemary, lavender, clove, cinnamon, myrrh and nutmeg. Other contributions to the development of aromatherapy were made by Conrad Gesner, and by Ryff, a Strasburg physician, who published his *Neu Gross Destillierbuch* in 1545.[15] The second official Nuremburg edition of the *Dispensatorium Valerii Cordi*, issued in 1592, lists sixty-one distilled essential oils. In his *Kräuterbuch*[16] Lonicer (1550) stressed the medicinal value of 'many marvellous and efficient oils of spices and seeds'.

H.B., in his *magnum opus* refers to *balsam oil*, although I am not certain which plant he means. He lists many uses for this oil including snake bite, scorpion bite, headache and fever. Myrrh oil is recommended for colds, wounds and insomnia, and saffron for 'keeping your head clear' if you are going to drink alcohol. Saffron oil was also rubbed on the head for a hangover, or into the chest to treat cardiac pain. It is a fascinating book and we see, perhaps for the first time since Avicenna, mention of essential oils being taken internally. Many books on distillation were written during the sixteenth century, especially in Germany, which seems to have been the centre of this aromatherapy renaissance. The books also frequently referred to alchemical practices. Alchemy was very popular at this time, and the distillation of all kinds of substances was one of the alchemists' favourite pastimes in their pursuit of the 'quintessence'* of matter.

In *The Treasure of Euonymus*, published in 1559,[17] Conrad Gesner speaks of essential oils having the power to 'conserve all strengths, and to prolong life'. His comments on the properties of rosemary oil are remarkably perceptive: 'It strengtheneth the harte, the braine, the sinnewes [muscles] and the hoole bodye . . . Members [limbs] sick of the palsy it heateth them for the mooste parte, and healeth them sometimes. Fistulaes and Cancars that give not place to other medicines, it healeth them throughlye.' Gesner was Swiss, probably knew H.B. and was a lifelong friend of William Turner, a famous English herbalist and botanist. Gesner's frequent handling of aromatics did not, sadly, prevent him dying from the first European Plague, which started in 1563.

Some of the important German works on distillation were translated into English, but had little impact until the following century. In *The Castel of Helth*,[18] published in 1541, Sir Thomas Elyot Knyght gives an amusing description of massage to stimulate the circulation: '. . . they do first softly, and afterward faster, rub their breaste and sydes downewarde, and overthwarte, not touching their stomake or bealy, and after cause their servant semblably to rubbe overthwarte their shulders and backe.' He goes on to say that the old infused-oil recipes, handed down from the Greeks and Romans, were rarely used, except for a few specific purposes. One gets the impression from this book that massage was not much used then, and that there was little awareness of its benefits.

* This word gave rise to 'essential oil'.

Just nineteen years before the publication of Braun-schweig's *New Vollkomen Distillierbuch*, a Chinese herbal text of major importance appeared. The *Pen Ts'ao*, or *Materia Medica*, of Li Shih-Chen[19] was the culmination of twenty-six years of writing and research, and covered almost 2000 herbs. The essential oils of twenty of these are described, including the following.

Essence of rose. This was said to act on the liver, stomach and blood, and was also employed as an anti-depressant.

Essence of jasmine. This was used as a general tonic for all the organs of the body.

Essence of white lotus flower. This was used as a remedy for coughs and for the coughing of blood from the lungs.

Essence of camomile. This was given for headaches, dizziness and colds.

Essence of ginger. This was used to treat mucousy coughs and malaria.

Many of these comments, especially the properties ascribed to rose oil, would be regarded as valid by modern aroma-therapists. Distillation was not known in China until a comparatively late date, but Shih-Chen's book is evidence that they were quick to incorporate aromatherapy into their traditional herbal practices.

The Seventeenth Century

This was the 'golden age' of English herbalists, notably Nicholas Culpeper, John Parkinson and John Gerarde. It was a time when the Plague returned with a vengeance, only to be outdone by the Great Fire of London in 1666. It was a time of pestilence, pomanders and yet more perfumes, although a few brave souls revived interest in the lost art of having a bath. By this time essential oils were becoming much more widely used, both by herbalists and doctors. In 1616 J. J. Wecker, a German, wrote: 'Perfumes are certainly compound medicaments, which without being heated can affect the mind, and eliminate all bad odours and infection in the air which surrounds us.' A very enlightened statement for 1616, and very pertinent to aromatherapy since all perfumes were made from natural essential oils.

The first popular perfume, 'Hungary water', had appeared in 1370. Based on rosemary oil, various stimulating and curative properties were ascribed to it. Since that time aromatic waters had been widely used, and many of them were distilled in monasteries. Carmelite balm water, for instance, was made by Carmelite monks from lemon balm (melissa) and other herbs. This was used by the monks as a remedy for various internal and external problems. Another popular 'perfume remedy' of the time was probably used as a cure-all, as it was called *Aqua Mirabilis* or 'miracle water'. A book of recipes, published in 1681, states that *Aqua Mirabilis* 'suffereth not the heat to burne nor melancholy nor flegme to be lift up or to have dominion above nature, it also expells reumes and profiteth a good colour, keepeth and preserveth visage and ye memory'.

The second visitation of the Plague came in 1603 and lasted up until the Great Fire of London in 1666. It so frightened people that for decades after remedies were touted as preventatives against the Black Death. At the time many things were tried, but the most popular and widely used were aromatics. It has been said that the perfumers of the period were immune because they were constantly surrounded by essential oils. A medical writer recommended 'such things as exhale very subtle sulphurs, as the spicy drugs and gums'. Among these he includes benzoin, styrax, frankincense and all aromatic woods and

roots. Master Alexis of Piedmont, a well-known alchemist
of the time, published a book with a number of pestilence
prophylactics, including: 'To make a verie good perfume
against the Plague, you must take Mastich, Chypre, Incense, Mace, Wormwood, Myrrh, Aloes Wood, Musk,
Ambergris, Nutmegs, Myrtle, Bay, Rosemary, Sage, Roses,
Elder, Cloves, Juniper, Rue and Pitch. All these things
stamped and mixed together, you shall set upon the coales
and so perfume the Chamber.' This recipe is obviously
based on the theory that the more aromatics you use, the
more likely you are to be successful, a concept which was
taken to even further extremes in the eighteenth century.
Many other aromatic recipes were proposed and indeed
were used to ward off the terrible infection, including cloves
of garlic, aromatic balls to hold in the hand and smell and
pomanders to carry about or hang up. We know that all
essential oils are antiseptic, and in fact there was nothing
better available to seventeenth-century man. There is no
way of judging how effective were the various aromatics
used, but it is quite feasible that many lives were saved by
such measures.

By the seventeenth century essential oils had become a
small but regular part of the herbalist's repertoire of
remedies. For instance, Culpeper (1653)[20] says of rosemary:
'The chymical [essential] oil drawn from the leaves and
flowers is a sovereign help . . . to touch the temples and
nostrils with two or three drops for all the diseases of the
head and brain spoken of before; as also to take one drop,
two or three, as the case requires, for the inward diseases;
yet it must be done with discretion, for it is very quick and
piercing.' An Englishman by the name of John Pechey
wrote a herbal in 1694[21] in which he is generally even more
enthusiastic than Culpeper about the benefits of essential
oils. Of clove oil he says: 'Oyl of cloves by Distillation is

good for inward and outward use. Some drops of it are, mixed with Cotton, put into aching Teeth. 'Tis likewise good in Malignant Fevers, and the Plague. The dose is two or three Drops in Balm-water, or some appropriate liquor.'

It is clear from these extracts that essential oils were already being used for a variety of internal and external problems. They were mainly used by herbalists, but also by doctors, a trend that was to continue until the end of the nineteenth century. They were still used very much less than herbs, but dosages had been established, the need for dilution and suitable vehicles for internal use had become clear and many of the healing properties were now well known. Aromatherapy had come a long way since the dark and superstitious Middle Ages, although it still had no clear identity and was not being used with massage, except on rare occasions.

The Eighteenth Century

During the eighteenth century essential oils were used by virtually all herbalists, and to an increasing degree by doctors. The apothecary was the predecessor of the modern pharmacist, and had originated from the physician's assistant, who would mix up the remedies for him. During the sixteenth century apothecaries became independent, and opened shops where the public could purchase remedies direct. Every apothecary had its own still, for preparing essential oils and aromatic waters. For the past few centuries these had also been in demand for mixing up magical oils for use in casting spells. This had its secretive and serious side (as it still does today) but also led to a demand, once the apothecary shops were established, for love potions and the like. These were largely based on aromatic oils and waters. Alchemists had also been hard at work for centuries, and embraced distillation with open arms when it became known. In fact there was such a close connection between distillation and alchemy that many people who wrote about, or used distillation were automatically labelled as alchemists, and the distinction between herbalist, chemist and alchemist was often indistinct.

Alchemists were generally perceived as being the most optimistic people, searching for the 'philosopher's stone' which would turn any metal into gold, and for the 'elixir of life'. They used distillation a great deal, not only for plants but for all kinds of substances; they made the whole process into a complex, mystical event, and occasionally blew themselves up in the fanatical pursuit of their goal. However, many of the early alchemists (there were no chemists as such then) made important chemical discoveries in their laboratories, and a seventeenth-century alchemist, Paracelsus, is credited with initiating interest in chemicals as drugs.[22] This led, from about 1650, to a gradual split between those physicians who increasingly used chemical drugs and those who remained faithful to herbs. The herbalists gradually fell from grace, which was precipitated by the now unfashionable association between herbal medicine and astrology. However, both groups continued to use essential oils.

The Nineteenth Century

During this century the medical doctor became well established as the family physician and, despite the relatively primitive transport situation, would visit as much as he was visited. Hence the birth of the 'doctor's bag' which contained all his standard remedies, including a few essential oils. William Whitla's *Materia Medica*,[23] first published in 1882, contains twenty-two official essential oils, and three unofficial ones. The official ones include camomile, cinnamon, fennel, juniper, bay, rosemary and thyme. In spite of their regular but relatively small use by doctors, essential oils never really caught on with the medical profession whose interest was firmly fixed on chemical drugs, and gradually essential oils were replaced by more 'reliable' remedies. This, curiously, coincided with the beginning of serious scientific tests and trials on essential oils.

Herbalists, as well as doctors, had taken to using essential oils less and less during the second half of the nineteenth century when, what was little more than a rumour, re-kindled the fire. Somebody drew attention to the low incidence of tuberculosis in the flower-growing districts of France. Tuberculosis was very much more common in those days, and France, especially in the south, had acres of flowers (now sadly gone) which were being grown for the expanding essential oil industry. It was also noted that most of the workers who processed the fragrant flowers and herbs remained quite free from respiratory diseases. The obvious cause of this was the essential oils contained in these plants. This led, in 1887, to the first recorded laboratory test on the anti-bacterial properties of essential oils. The role of micro-organisms in disease had only been recognized seven years before.

Chamberland, in Paris, in 1887,[24] and Cadéac and Meunier, in 1888, published similar studies which showed that the micro-organisms of glanders and yellow fever were easily killed by essential oils. The most effective ones were cinnamon, thyme, lavender, juniper, sandalwood and cedarwood. Since that time a great many tests have been performed in the laboratory on the anti-bacterial and anti-fungal effects of essential oils. It is a huge subject, which I cannot cover here, and it seems very strange that the more tests that were done on essential oils the less they were being used by the medical profession. By the 1940s their recognized medicinal applications had virtually been reduced to the role of flavouring agents for real medicines. Laboratory testing does have certain drawbacks, which eventually led to the development of a new type of test now used by French aromatherapy doctors, called the *aromatogram* (see page 74).

The Twentieth Century

The case for aromatherapy, however, is not confined to laboratory testing. In an article for the *Practitioner* in 1918[25] an English doctor, W. Minchin, wrote: 'There is probably no more valuable drug mentioned in any pharmacopoeia than *oleum alii* [garlic oil] the active principle of garlic; yet there is scarcely any so little known to our profession generally.' He had been investigating and using garlic for nearly twenty years, and had found it an effective treatment for tuberculosis (TB), lupus and especially for diphtheria, which, like TB, was often fatal. He realized that, unlike any other known antiseptics, garlic was completely harmless to the body tissue. In his article Minchin quotes a clinical trial conducted at the Metropolitan Hospital in New York, when fifty-six modern treatments were tried over two years on 1082 TB patients. Every known therapy was included – vaccines, serums, antitoxins, surgery, arsenic and mercury compounds and garlic. The hospital report concluded: 'Garlic gave us our best results, and would seem equally efficacious, no matter what part of the body was affected.'

It was a French cosmetic chemist, Réné-Maurice

Gattefossé, who coined the term 'aromatherapy' in 1937. He used the word as the title for his book, published in that year,[26] which was mainly concerned with the anti-microbial effects of the oils. Between the first study in 1887, and 1937, fifty years later, over a hundred journal articles had been published on this subject. Neither these, nor clinical trials like the one in New York, did anything to persuade the medical profession at large that essential oils had any real use apart from that of flavouring agents. Gattefossé spoke of aromatherapy as 'a therapy employing aromatics in a sphere of research opening enormous vistas to those who have started exploring it'. He was very interested in the application of aromatherapy for skin problems, both cosmetic and medical. He discovered the effectiveness of lavender oil on burns, after injuring his hand in a small laboratory explosion and subsequently treating it with the oil. The effect of lavender oil on burns remains one of the most miraculous, and yet unexploited, phenomena of aromatherapy.

Although Gattefossé deserves full credit for his vision of aromatherapy, he was not the only one at that time to recognize and investigate the benefits of essential oils. In 1939 another Frenchman, Albert Couvreur, published a book on the medicinal applications of essential oils.[27] In Australia Penfold and others were discovering the benefits of tea-tree oil, while in Italy two doctors, Giovanni Gatti and Renato Cayola, were delving into the psychotherapeutic applications of essential oils. Many other lone researchers, mostly unaware of the growing evidence for aromatherapy as a whole, contributed their own efforts in countries as far apart as Japan, the USA, the USSR and the UK. Just one of many unsung pioneers was a certain Dr H. Sztark, French medical inspector of schools in the late 1930s. Influenced by Gattefossé, he introduced vaporization of a mixture of essential oils to every school he visited, for use in all class-rooms. This, he wrote, had a dual purpose: 'Odeur agréable dans les classes et désinfectant par excellence.' (Being both volatile and antiseptic, essential oils are the ideal means of preventing the spread of airborne infection.)

The Second World War brought the progress of aromatherapy to a standstill, with one notable exception. A certain Dr Jean Valnet, an army surgeon, had also been greatly influenced by the work of Gattefossé, and he used essential oils as antiseptics in the treatment of war wounds, which it was his job to sew up. After the war he continued using the oils in his capacity as a doctor, and in 1964 published a comprehensive work[28] entitled *Aromathérapie* (now available in English), which has since earned him global recognition. Shortly after this he began teaching other doctors about the healing benefits of essential oils. There are now at least four establishments in France where medical doctors can learn aromatherapy, and some 1500 general practitioners now prescribe essential oils. Let us hope that doctors in other countries follow this excellent example.

A number of doctors and researchers have made valuable contributions to aromatherapy during the last twenty to thirty years, notably Professor Paolo Rovesti of Milan University in Italy. However, we cannot end this story without acknowledging the very special contribution of Marguerite Maury. She practised and taught aromatherapy until her death in 1964, and wrote two books on the subject. The second, *Le Capital 'Jeunesse'*,[29] was translated into English as *The Secret of Life and Youth* (now sadly out of print), a title which accurately reflects the book's preoccupation with rejuvenation. She does not give very much practical information, but must have been a very gifted, and visionary person. She recognized the value of ancient teachings, and writes about traditional Hindu, Chinese and Tibetan medicine, and their various philosophies. She conceived the notion of the 'individual prescription', a simple blend of essential oils that would operate on more than the physical level and would normalize the unbalanced functions in the whole person. And, most importantly, she realized the significance of applying the oils *externally*, diluted in vegetable oil, in combination with massage. She was seeking for an alternative method to oral application, which she was not happy with, and devotes a whole chapter in her book to finding this alternative method. She writes: 'Gattefossé spoke of a cutaneous application, of a penetration through the skin, but how? Under what conditions?' It may seem obvious and simple to us now, but, until she reintroduced the concept, essential oils had not been used in combination with massage for almost 1000 years, with a few exceptions. The word *holistic* had not been coined in her day, but it was Marguerite Maury who revived the ancient art of what we now call holistic aromatherapy.

CHAPTER THREE

HOW IT WORKS

Aromatherapy . . . is not just *another medicine*, a heretical and unofficial one. On the contrary, it has come through experimental method to occupy its rightful place among the most effective remedies in therapeutic use.

Paolo Rovesti

Holism – the Key to Healing

After 'What is aromatherapy?' the two questions I am asked most frequently are: 'How does it work?' and 'What proof is there?' I hope this chapter answers these questions fairly, and with as few complexities as possible. To spotlight the way in which essential oils work let us make a simple analogy between them and chemical drugs. Essential oils are extremely complex substances, chemically speaking, and their effects on the body are both complex and subtle. If we imagine that healing is like opening a door, the action of a chemical drug is like that of a sledge-hammer, while the action of an essential oil is like that of a key. The key is apparently much less powerful – it is very much smaller, and it is more difficult to demonstrate its effectiveness. However, the key works very much 'in harmony' with the nature of the door; in fact the door-lock was made to receive a key. In opening the door the key proves its usefulness without the destructive, harmful effects of the sledge-hammer. However, keys have one drawback. While a sledge-hammer will open any door, the key will only work *if you use the correct key for the individual lock.* The 'key' is equivalent to the correct blend of essential oils and massage. We could add that the best way to demonstrate the effectiveness of the key is to simply open the door – to show that people are healed by aromatherapy.

To take this analogy a little further we could say that, even if we have the right key, if we do not apply it correctly, by putting it into the lock, the door will not open. In aromatherapy the massage is like placing the key, directing the essential oils and the patient's body to interact in a certain way. If you make up a blend of essential oils for someone and then just show them the bottle, or allow them only to smell it, you will not achieve anything like the same results as if you apply the oils along with the appropriate massage. It goes further still. The *right* essential oils and the *wrong* massage, or the *right* massage and the *wrong* essential oils, will not give positive results. You need the right key *and* you need to put it in the lock. The impetus to turn the key and push the door open is provided by the patient/therapist interplay, based on trust and sound advice. Without the desire for health, and the momentum of feeling better and making progress, the heavier doors will not open.

It may take time to get the door open. Maybe it has been closed for many years, and not everyone is prepared for the implications of healing, of going through the door and facing up to what is on the other side. This is one reason why an understanding and experienced therapist is so valuable. The right kind of reassurance will go a long way, and when the key starts to turn and the door starts to move it always feels right, even if it is a little uncomfortable at times. In some ways sickness is a result of failure to cope with a life situation. The one I come across most frequently is the married woman in her forties, with children in their mid-teens. After twenty or so years of marriage she is wondering if she still loves her husband and if she wants to spend the rest of her life with him. There are no natural remedies for life situations as such, but we can come very close to it by using essential oils which aid clarity, help boost self-confidence or uplift the spirits. We all encounter problem situations involving relationships, work, money or health, and aromatherapy can help us to cope with them because of its therapeutic effects on the psyche.

George Bernard Shaw once defined a specialist as someone who 'learns more and more about less and less until ultimately he knows everything about nothing'. Anyone who has delved very deeply into a subject will recognize the truth of this statement. The nature of all scientific research is such that it is constrained to follow exactly this path. It is an approach to finding the 'truth' proposed by the philosopher Descartes, and is known as *reductionism* because it involves a process of narrowing down, or reducing. Facts are analysed in fine detail, chemicals are purified to the nth degree, and the microscope increases its power until a point is reached where matter no longer exists. Reductionism is an integral part of the way we all think and act. It has innumerable uses, and I am certainly not criticizing scientific research – much of the evidence for aromatherapy in these pages comes from such research. However, natural therapists do not practise their therapy purely on the basis of research and scientific 'proof'. This is one of the basic differences between conventional and non-conventional medicine. We do recognize the value of science, but we also have other values – first, *empiricism* – what works, works, and if we do not have a 'scientific' explanation that is no reason to reject it out of hand. Second, we have certain philosophical values, or beliefs, which might be labelled as 'esoteric'.

Conventional medicine has become in most areas, a slave to the reductionist philosophy. One result is that it can teach us a tremendous amount about our bodies and about disease, but not so much about healing. The therapeutics of conventional medicine have been left far too much in the hands of the pharmaceutical companies. The widespread use of pure, chemical drugs is another natural consequence of too much reductionism. Many plants have had their 'active principle' extracted, or manufactured synthetically, to give us drugs like atropine (belladonna), digitalis (foxglove) or aspirin (willow). Strangely this fact is sometimes used by the medical profession to give drug therapy a more wholesome image. The 'active principle' principle is a flawed one. It is rather like eating a vitamin C tablet instead of an orange, or a vitamin A capsule instead of a carrot. Nutritionists now recognize that other elements also have to be present for one vitamin or mineral to be properly absorbed by the body. Coming back to aromatherapy, we find that the major constituent of an essential oil may be more active for one or two functions only, but is invariably *less* active than the natural oil in every other way. As we have already seen, power is not everything; safety and subtlety must also be considered.

It seems to be the nature of chemical drugs that they have side-effects. Almost as a penalty for their guaranteed action on one level, something goes wrong on another. Drug-induced disease, known as *iatrogenic* disease, is thought to account for at least 15 per cent of all illnesses today. Natural remedies rarely cause such problems, if ever, because they are highly complex, organic substances. The ingredients of such a remedy function in harmony with each other, and in harmony with the human organism, rather than against it. Essential oils consist of, on average, 100 different chemicals, some of them in extremely small amounts. It is feasible that each one of those minor constituents performs some useful function, which partly would explain why essential oils are useful in so many different conditions. Because they are complex, essential oils also work on many different levels, affecting body chemistry, nervous function, digestive function, mood and so on.

An example of the fallacy of isolating the 'active principle' can be seen in the essential oil of lemongrass. The major constituent of this oil is an aldehyde *citral*, which is present at a level of around 80 per cent. If the citral is extracted from the oil (or made synthetically) and applied to the skin it will cause an allergic reaction. However, lemongrass oil does not cause such a reaction. This puzzled toxicologists, who were testing perfume ingredients for skin reactions. They designed a further test which showed conclusively that other constituents in the natural oil somehow buffer the potentially hazardous effect of the citral.[1] Natural remedies, most of which have been in use for centuries, do not give rise to the type of side-effects associated with drug therapy. It is true that some essential oils are toxic. Bitter almond oil, for instance, contains a 3 per cent level of prussic acid (cyanide) in its natural state, but of course the oil is never used until all the cyanide has been removed. Most almond flavourings are now made from synthetically manufactured *benzaldehyde*, which constitutes the other 97 per cent of the natural oil. The toxic oils are not used in aromatherapy, although they could feasibly be useful in homoeopathic doses.

Conventional medicine has lost much of its previous close contact with patients, and in some ways is becoming increasingly technologized and dehumanized. Paradoxically there is, at the same time, an increasing awareness among many doctors (especially the younger ones) of the benefits of complementary therapies. This awareness is also growing among physiotherapists and nurses, who have more direct contact with patients, and who are beginning to take an active interest in massage, reflexology and aromatherapy. Viewpoints are changing rapidly, and natural therapists are also recognizing that conventional medicine has its good points. Chemical drugs can save lives in critical circumstances, but they are grossly overprescribed for a host of relatively minor complaints which, in the long run, might be better treated with the use of natural remedies. In a great many cases the patient would benefit if complementary therapy was the first resort, instead of the last. The trend in the UK is certainly in that direction and, after 300 years of divergence, conventional and complementary medicine have begun to re-merge.

There is no universally accepted definition of holism. Some say that it means practising several different therapies and must include a knowledge of diet and nutrition. Others feel that the practice of one therapy is sufficient, as long as 'the whole person' is considered – mind, body and soul. Let us remember that there is a fundamental difference between the reductionist and holistic philosophies. One is based on experiment, and the other on empiricism (what is found to work). Another difference in philosophy involves the concept of 'life force'. According to the reductionist theory this does not exist, since it has not been scientifically measured or otherwise analysed. Medical science does not embrace concepts of subtle, healing energies.

Healing Energies

The concept of life force, or subtle energy, is a very old one. The Chinese call it *chi*, the Japanese *ki*, and the Indians *prana*. All living things have a non-physical life energy. We have it, plants have it, and natural essential oils have it. There are such things as 'reconstituted essential oils' which are made by putting together the same chemical constituents as are found in the real thing. They are, of course, cheaper, but often smell noticeably different, and do not have the same therapeutic capacity and integrity as the natural oils. Some vital ingredient, a non-chemical one, is missing. Admittedly it is almost impossible to duplicate natural oils even chemically, because they have so many constituents present in extremely small amounts, as low as 0·00001 per cent. However, even if we could get around that problem, I doubt whether the result would match up to nature's manufacturing genius. There is more to life than chemistry, and essential oils, though not alive in the normal sense, undoubtedly have some subtle healing energy.

Essential oils are positively pro-life and pro-health. We know, for instance, that they are able to stimulate tissue regeneration. In the case of skin burns, lavender, and other oils stimulate the growth of new healthy skin, resulting in very rapid healing.[2,3] The stimulating effect of essential oils on the healing process can also be witnessed in the rapid healing of wounds, sores and ulcers, even in cases which have failed to respond to other treatments. Bone tissue regeneration may also be stimulated by essential oils, evidenced by their success in treating osteoporosis/arthritis and in speeding the healing of broken bones (see p. 99). Tissue regeneration in the livers of rats has been demonstrated with essential oils, in particular the four seed oils cumin, fennel, celery and parsley.[4]

We know that essential oils stimulate the immune system (scc p. 78), partly by stimulating the production of white blood cells. The regeneration of skin tissue, mentioned above, must be due to an invigoration of cell activity and growth. Since ageing involves a slowing down of cell renewal there is some basis for the claim that aromatherapy is 'rejuvenating', although I would much prefer to call it 'health preserving'. In 1559 Conrad Gesner referred to essential oils as having the power to conserve health and to prolong youth.

Several sources mention the electrical aspect of aromatherapy and cell stimulation. Rovesti states that the electromagnetic charge of the aromatic molecules of essential oils has 'a sharp influence on cellular magnetic fields'.[5] Valnet refers to the electrical resistance of essential oils.[3] He makes the point that cancer is a condition in which the electrical resistance of cells is reduced, and that clove oil, which has a high resistance, displays anticarcinogenic properties. He also comments that the high resistance of essences discourages the diffusion of infections and toxins.

For centuries it has been claimed that all living things are surrounded by an 'aura'. This is a field of energy extending beyond the limits of the physical body. I do not doubt the existence of auras, since I am lucky enough to be able to see them. Most people find this difficult, but feeling the subtle energy around someone's body is relatively easy and many people could learn to do this. In the USA, Dolores Krieger, Professor of Nursing at New York University, teaches this technique to nurses, and has written a book called *The Therapeutic Touch*.[6] Psychic healing is of course nothing new, and is based on the principle of 'energizing' the patient's subtle energy 'body', or healing it in some way.

Some years ago a Russian scientist, Semyon Kirlian, developed a method of photographing the 'aura'. This technique uses ordinary photographic paper, but, instead of a camera, an instrument which produces a high-voltage electrical field is used. Anything which is alive, whether plant or animal, shows an energy field around it when photographed in this way. Many of those who use this technique are trying to demystify it, pointing out, quite correctly, that it does not show the aura as such, but rather an electrical effect of the auric field. A form of diagnosis/analysis has recently been evolved based on Kirlian photographs of patients' hands (see Figure 2).

The Importance of Touch

There is quite a body of evidence now pointing to the fact that being touched is an essential component of optimum health, and in early life it is vital.[7] Baby animals need to be licked by their mothers shortly after birth. If this does not happen for any reason they usually die, unless their skin is stimulated by some other means. (Mother and baby also learn to recognize each other by smell within an hour of birth. Human babies learn their mother's unique scent, within six weeks of birth.) During the nineteenth century a great many children died of a disease called *marasmus*, the medical term for 'wasting away'. This can be caused by extreme malnutrition, but in many cases was due to lack of love, and most of these deaths occurred in children's institutions and orphanages. In 1915 a New York pediatrician reported that all children under the age of two died when put into an institution. This was later ascribed to the fact that these babies were not handled or loved in any way, in accordance with the advice of many nineteenth-century

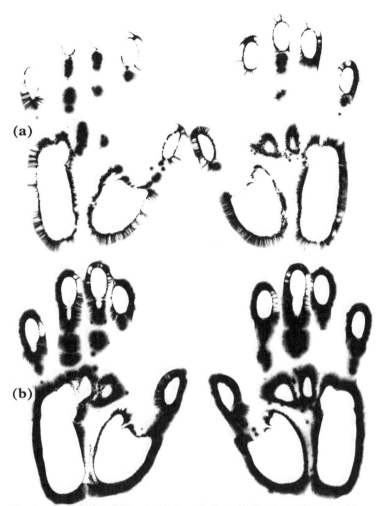

Figure 2. Kirlian photographs of the hands of a forty-seven-year-old female patient. (a) Before treatment. At this time she was going through a period of great emotional stress and was trying to come off tranquillizers. Both hands indicate several stress areas. (b) After a full-body aromatherapy massage with oils of lavender, lemongrass and basil. There is an overall increase in energy radiation. Stress areas, though still evident, are reducing. (Photograph courtesy of Rosemary Steel)

pediatricians who strongly advised against 'fussing'. Love is communicated to babies largely through the sense of touch, and a severe lack of it can be fatal. It was not until the 1930s that a policy of 'mothering' was introduced into hospitals and homes caring for young children. In the Bellevue Hospital in New York this resulted in a reduction in infant mortality from 35 per cent to less than 10 per cent by 1938.

There have been a number of studies on animals which show that handling (by humans) in early life leads to a more emotionally stable and unexcitable animal. In his excellent book *Touching*[7] Dr Ashley Montagu comments on these studies, including one in which the thyroid gland was removed from 304 rats.[8] Of those which had not been handled when young, 79 per cent died, but of those which had been handled only 13 per cent died. Dr Montagu remarks: 'Gentle handling of rats could make all the difference between life and death following the removal of significant endocrine glands. This discovery was striking enough, but what was equally remarkable was the influence of gentling on behavioural development. Gentling produced gentle, unexcitable animals; lack of gentling resulted in fearful, agitated animals.' In another experiment with rats the level of certain vital body chemicals, including growth hormone, was shown to decrease after pups were removed from their mothers.[9] In a further study, one group (the control group) of rat pups remained with mum, while two other groups were removed and stroked with a soft brush. One group was stroked lightly, and the other heavily. This last group, which experienced skin stimulation similar to gentle handling, or massage, showed no change, as did the control group. (The group that was stroked lightly showed significant reductions in growth hormone levels, and in brain, heart and liver activity.)[10] Many other studies give further evidence for the fact that skin stimulation, or touching, is one of the most vital ingredients of early life. Apart from nutrition it is perhaps the most vital.

Human babies thrive best if they are touched and loved frequently, and also if they are talked to, sung to and carried around close to mother or father. In an unpublished study Weininger reported that infants whose backs were stroked by their mothers from ten weeks of age had fewer problems from catarrh, colds, vomiting and diarrhoea than babies who were not stroked. More recently it has been found that premature babies in hospital incubators are more likely to thrive and survive if handled daily. This practice stemmed from the experience of a maternity hospital in Bogotá, Colombia, which could not afford the luxury of incubators for premature babies. It was noticed that they survived very well in a sling placed between their mothers' breasts.[11]

Those who suffered a lack of loving/touching when young are said to have a disproportionate need to be touched in adult life, and this is often a contributing factor in emotional problems. Women who are not loved/touched sufficiently by their husbands often use the sexual act as a means of attracting the loving touch they really need. Dr Montagu comments: 'There are significant biochemical differences between humans who have enjoyed adequate tactile stimulation and those who have not, a statement that will probably be found to hold true throughout life: that the unloved person, taken at any age, is likely to be a very different biochemical entity from those who have been adequately loved.'

In a study at Purdue University, Indiana, in 1986, students who took out books from the library were interviewed as they came out. They were asked specific questions relating to their opinion of the library and whether the check-out assistant had smiled at them. The library assistant treated everyone in exactly the same way, except that every other student was lightly touched on the hand as their library card was handed back to them. Those who were touched formed a more positive view of the library than those who were not and often thought that the assistant had smiled at them, although in fact she had not.

Massage

Massage is possibly the only situation in which we can be touched in a caring way by someone who is not close to us, and not worry about it. The question which naturally arises from the previous discussion, then, is can this in any way compensate for problems stemming from not being adequately touched/loved when we were young? Or from not being lovingly touched as adults? There are no experimental studies to guide us here, but I think the answer would have to be yes, to some extent. Exactly to what extent I cannot say, but would draw the reader's attention to the survey summarized in Table 1 (p. 6) which shows that a high percentage (82 per cent) of people who had massage felt they had benefited from it.

It would be interesting to find out whether people who feel adequately *loved* still have a great need for touch. In our culture touching is taboo in many situations, and yet it may be that simply being touched somehow makes us feel loved. Loving and touching are so closely related; witness expressions like 'He touched my heart' or 'I felt really touched'. Massage is not all caresses, much of it involves some degree of discomfort, and yet people do not mind this at all if it is done in the right way. You can cause someone pain by hitting them, and you can relieve pain that people sometimes do not even know they have by releasing muscular tension. Both hurting and healing can feel painful, but somehow it is a quite different type of pain. An ache that feels good might be a better way of describing it.

The physical benefits of massage are quite comprehensive. It stimulates the circulation of blood and lymph, reduces high blood pressure, stimulates the immune system, reduces muscular tension, reduces swelling and relieves pain in muscles and joints. For many people massage is the most important aspect of an aromatherapy treatment, because they find it so soothing and revitalizing. Sometimes patients do fall asleep on the treatment couch, but deep relaxation does not have to lead to sleep, and can be achieved without it. Some people are more refreshed after a good massage than after a night's sleep – even in sleep muscles can remain in a state of tension. However, in the long term massage does improve the quality of sleep and the degree of relaxation. More than once a patient has returned for their second treatment to announce that, the night of the first one, they slept better than they had done for years.

This kind of relaxation is a feature of body-contact therapies, as opposed to prescription therapies. It is one reason for their growing popularity, and its importance in the healing process should not be underestimated. The simple act of massaging and relaxing muscles encourages the mind to take a break from its usual frenetic activity. Muscular tension is often directly related to psychological tension and repressed emotions. The act of soothing the physical tension has a reflex effect on the psychological tension and so helps to break down what is known as 'armouring' – the barriers and defences we build between us and the outside world. There does not have to be any emotional outburst for tension to be released. Feelings are often 'brought to the surface' by massage, which occasionally results in a few tears and often to talking out problems. This demonstrates the emotionally releasing effects of massage, but just as often it is a quiet, pleasant and tearless affair.

A good massage, like anything which has a deeply relaxing effect, is followed by a feeling of well-being and an increase in our general energy level. We could say that energies which were being blocked by tension have now been allowed to flow normally, and so naturally we experience more energy. Tension traps energy, relaxation releases it. If tiredness is the first indication of ill health, then massage should be the first resort.

Our need to be loved/touched is greater when we are seriously stressed or ill. In *The Transparent Self*[12] Jourard suggests that touch can alleviate stress and by doing so enable the patient to mobilize their own healing potential. Massage is already being used in some hospitals to relieve muscle tension, promote sleep, relieve pain and reduce high blood pressure, as well as for its comforting effect. Plaxy Kinney, a nurse in the Oxford Nursing Development Unit in the Radcliffe Infirmary, comments: 'As well as for sedation, massage with essential oils is often used as an alternative to analgesia, particularly for the kinds of pain not easily dealt with by tablets and injections, like stump pains of a "phantom" nature. Nurses will sometimes pass on massage and the use of essential oils to patients' relatives.'

In a recent study[13] Sally Sims, nursing lecturer at King's College, London, investigated the value of massage in the general care of cancer patients. Six women with breast cancer were given a gentle, soft-tissue back massage for ten minutes, using an unscented vegetable oil. Each of them received a total of six daily massages. A number of patient responses were measured, including mood, concentration, fatigue, nausea and pain. Results were compared to those of a control group, where patients laid down and rested for ten minutes. It was found that massage led to a significant improvement in fatigue and concentration. Both of these factors deteriorated by 25 per cent in the control group, but improved by 25 per cent following massage. This would seem to indicate that lying down does not necessarily lead to a restful state and supports my own claim that massage leads to an increase in energy levels. It was noted that four of the six patients started to talk about their personal concerns after their massage, showing that they had begun to 'let go'. It was also found that the patients generally felt better after massage: 'Results . . . indicate that patients reported less symptom distress, a higher degree of tranquillity and vitality, and less tension and tiredness following the slow stroke back massage.'

Aromatherapy is being used in the Compton Hospice, Wolverhampton, for the benefit of cancer patients. Mrs Kensey, Director of Nursing Services, explains: 'Cancer patients suffer from physical, mental, spiritual and social pain. Many patients have lived in isolation through the ignorance of family and friends, who are afraid to touch them. We have found great changes taking place in patients who have gone through this, by the fact that through gentle massage with oils and herbs they have been helped to relax, which has eased the physical pain and they have become less tense. Patients tend to open up and say what they are feeling and what their fears are. This in turn has enabled us to counsel patients far more easily and deal with psychological pain as well as social and physical pain. Patients with bone and muscular pain have benefited greatly from massage, and are able to move their limbs much more freely.

We often wonder how we ever coped without the aid of aromatherapy.'

We now have some real evidence that massage decreases stress in stressed adults (nobody with personal experience of professional massage would require any further evidence of its de-stressing effect). Dr Peter Nixon, consultant cardiologist at the Charing Cross Hospital, London, has introduced massage as part of a scheme to reduce stress in heart patients. Again, soft-tissue massage is used, as part of a programme to rehabilitate patients in whom stress has caused a severe deterioration of health. Nixon explains: 'Patients with various heart conditions are massaged and, if this leads to improvement through fall of blood pressure and emotional tension, for example, the patient is given the chance to improve upon this by his or her own efforts, which will be guided by the therapist. The massage helps to establish a good relationship and this encourages the patient to follow the advice of the therapist and to take every opportunity for self-help.'

A report in *Disability Now*,[15] the journal of the Spastics Society, reveals that seven women at a care centre in Oxford have adopted aromatherapy. The aromatherapist, who visits them regularly, comments: 'One thing – more than anything else – stood out as the group developed: the need to be touched.' These disabled women have found that aromatherapy helps them with a number of individual problems; P M S, for instance, can be so much worse if you are also disabled. However, they all find that it helps in three common problem areas: poor circulation, nervous tension and lack of self-esteem. The group's secretary states: 'One of my main aims is to promote massage and aromatherapy because they really do help us.' The physical contact of the massage, and the uplifting effect of the essential oils, help them to feel more confident and relaxed, and so enriches their experience of life. There are times in all of our lives when we have a similar need, especially if we have recently experienced divorce or bereavement.

Some of the major organs of the body, notably the large intestine, are accessible to massage. More deeply seated organs, such as the liver or kidneys, can be influenced by massage over the area of the body where they are situated. Sluggish or ailing organs are gently stimulated through increased local blood circulation and stimulation of nerve supply. More refined types of massage make use of pressure points, sometimes called 'trigger' points, which stimulate specific internal organs, even though these points may be some distance from the related organs.[14] The correct type of pressure, when applied to such trigger points, will 'energize' the appropriate organ by what is known as a 'reflex' effect (hence the term *reflexology*, which works on hand and foot reflexes). Such methods include acupressure and shiatsu (both based on acupuncture points) and neuromuscular massage, 'touch for health' (a form of muscle testing) and reflexology (based on other systems). At least one of these forms of pressure-point massage is normally used in aromatherapy, and all are disciplines in their own right, requiring specialized training. Some pressure-point techniques could be described as a link between a purely physical treatment and one which works on subtle energy imbalances.

While on the subject of massage, I should explain that both vegetable oils and essential oils are readily absorbed by human skin.[16,17] This is due partly to the volatile, semigaseous nature of essential oils and partly to the fact that they are lipids. Water-soluble substances get through the skin with very much more difficulty because it is basically waterproof.

Aromatherapy and Stress

Self-treatment can never be as beneficial as receiving an aromatherapy treatment from a skilled therapist. Even if you manage to hit on the right blend of essential oils, you cannot lie down, relax and be massaged by yourself. Aromatherapy without massage is rather like an orchestra without a conductor. The massage, in addition to its other benefits, is necessary to give direction to the treatment. The therapist orchestrates the treatment proceedings by talking to the patient's body with his or her hands: by encouraging oil absorption in key areas, by stimulating or relaxing where needed and sometimes by applying different oils to different parts of the body. A good body therapist has talking hands, a magic touch, which gently and purposefully encourage the healing process. A skilled therapist does not give everyone the same treatment, and oils need to be changed to suit the needs of each patient. During a treatment the therapist will adapt to the patient's needs, developing the massage as appropriate.

Essential oils and massage have much in common. Both can be relaxing and reduce stress; both can be stimulating and pain-relieving; both can lower blood pressure and stimulate the immune system; both can help to relieve muscular aches and other forms of distress such as period pains or headaches.

The power of aromatherapy lies in combining the two, and perhaps the one thing that aromatherapy is best known for is in counteracting stress, and the many conditions in which it plays a part, probably accounting for around 90 per cent of all health problems. How does it do this? One simple way of looking at it is shown in Figure 3. The 'stress cycle' is a vicious circle, a downward spiral. Four signs, or symptoms are shown, which are often the first indications

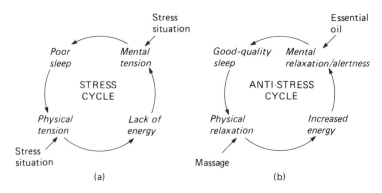

Figure 3. (a) Stress cycle; (b) anti-stress cycle.

that something is wrong – mental tension, poor sleep, physical tension and lack of energy. Other such warning signs may include pain, lack of appetite, irritability and a host of others. Signs such as these are part of everyday life for most of us, and when we can cope with them adequately there is no reason for alarm. It is when things start to get worse that we need to seek help, when our own stress cycle starts to control us and to make inroads into our wellbeing. There comes a point where we can no longer help ourselves, because our stress situation is more than we can handle, whether it is our own doing or quite beyond our control. Such a breakdown does not have to be dramatic, like a heart attack; it can be a very gradual slide, almost imperceptible.

I do not wish to imply that aromatherapy is the only solution to stress. There are many possible solutions, and we should also do everything possible to help ourselves. But most of us need help once we get stuck in a ditch. We need a tug from someone else to help haul us out. In terms of aromatherapy the tug might only take one treatment, or it might take twenty treatments; it all depends on how deeply we have sunk. How can aromatherapy help? As we can see in the diagram, essential oils work on the mental tension, while massage works on the physical tension. This is an oversimplification, but gives a fair idea of the reality. Once mental tension is relieved then sleep improves, which in turn relieves the physical tension. Once physical tension is eased then energy levels increase, and so we feel better, we are more relaxed and alert.

An improvement in these very common signs is the first thing I look for in a patient with a stress-related condition. Invariably such improvements are noticeable after only one treatment. Patients frequently offer comments to the effect that they are feeling better in themselves, they are sleeping better, are feeling less tired, their appetite or sex life has improved, or they are feeling generally brighter and more energetic. Aromatherapy does tend to make us feel good, if not during the treatment, then certainly afterwards. The reasons for this are complex, but it is in part due to the release of certain mood-inducing chemicals in the brain and body. These are known as *neurochemicals* because they interrelate with the nervous system. One, *noradrenaline*, is probably triggered by stimulating oils, and another, *serotonin*, by sedative oils.* Others, the *endorphins* and *enkephalins* are partly what make us feel good after a treatment. They are known to have a dual effect. One, you feel great, quietly euphoric, and two, they act as natural pain-killers. Soldiers horribly wounded in battle sometimes feel no pain for a while because their body releases a flood of analgesic neurochemicals. A study performed at the Peking Medical College showed that finger pressure on acupuncture

---

* Michael Shipley, a neurophysiologist at Cincinnati University, has demonstrated that fibres from the olfactory nerves carry impulses to two small but significant parts of the brain, the *locus ceruleus* (LC) and the *raphe nucleus* (RN): *Noradrenaline* is concentrated in the L C and *serotonin* in the R N.[18]

points could induce a rise in pain thresholds of up to 133 per cent due to an increase in the levels of endorphins and enkephalins.[19]

Pain and stress are very much related. Although none of the essential oils are thought to be very strong pain-killers, there are many conditions involving pain in which aroma-therapy has been known to bring relief. Examples include scorpion bites, poisonous spider bites, bee and wasp stings, neuralgia, sciatica, toothache and headache. The case histories in the following chapter also include several painful conditions – broken finger, sprained ankle, arthritis, period pains, sinusitis and earache. It seems likely that essential oils do not have a direct pain-killing effect, but act indirectly, by stimulating the release of the body's own natural analgesics.

Natural Balance

Every moment there are thousands of different actions taking place within your body for the purpose of maintaining a state of balance. The process of maintaining this state of harmony is known as *homeostasis*, and it involves every organ and function in the body. One obvious example is body temperature, which is largely affected by external conditions. If we did not have a built-in thermostat our body temperature would go up or down whenever the ambient temperature changed or whenever we had a hot or cold drink. Various warning signs protect us from other types of imbalance. Thirst protects us from dehydration, hunger from starvation, and fatigue from exhaustion. Many more subtle processes have to take place, unseen and largely unfelt by us, to maintain homeostasis. However, when homeostasis breaks down at some level, and when we ignore the small warning signals and continue as before, some form of illness is the usual result. Suppressing the warning sign or *symptom* with drugs is not usually sufficient to regain balance, what we call *health*.

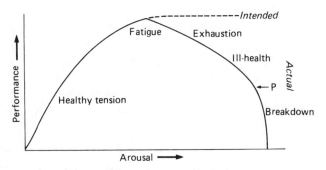

Figure 4. Breakdown (P) of therapeutic balance.

People who constantly ignore warning signs of fatigue, and who push themselves beyond their natural limits in their work, can overtax their hearts. Nixon uses the diagram illustrated in Figure 4 to highlight this situation. Performance and arousal (tension) are, within certain limits, normal and healthy. If we constantly push ourselves beyond the point of fatigue we court danger in the form of exhaustion, ill health and breakdown, which could be emotional or physical (e.g. heart attack). Nixon comments: 'Exhaustion with rage and despair is particularly dangerous from the homeostasis point of view. The commonest immediate causes seem to be ... people-poisoning; excessive time pressures; and resentment about changes imposed by others. The usual response is to deny the problems or reject them, and to press on regardless ... These vicious circles cannot be carried on indefinitely. Sooner or later homeostasis is violated, and malfunctions ultimately capable of causing a breakdown [at P in Figure 4] are set in train because the constancy of the internal milieu cannot be maintained.'[20] One of the commonest signs of ill health seen within this scheme is high blood pressure, and one of the tools Nixon employs in dealing with this is massage.

This same model could be applied to any illness situation, not just cardiovascular disease. It illustrates very clearly the role which the patients themselves often play, and of course the importance of not violating homeostasis, or natural balance. In other situations it will not be high blood pressure and heart attacks which ensue, but perhaps food allergies, colitis, P M S or eczema.

It would be fair to say that homeostasis is principally governed by the nervous and endocrine systems, and both can be influenced by many factors, including emotions and aromatherapy. Any therapy aims, directly or indirectly, to maintain or regain homeostasis. Through the nervous and endocrine systems every emotional and physical response can be triggered off. The influence of aromatherapy here can be seen in both massage and in essential oils. Nixon's work demonstrates that massage is capable of reducing blood pressure, and massage has an obvious influence on mood, tending to induce a state of relaxation and counteracting the effects of stress. The influence of essential oils here can be described in a little more detail.

In *Une Médecine nouvelle, phytothérapie et aromathérapie*[21] Valnet and co-authors list a number of essential oils which have particular effects on the autonomic nervous system and on the secretion of adrenaline and oestrogen. Oils of basil, pine and savory are said to stimulate the sympathetic nerves (i.e. they are stimulating) and they are also adrenal stimulants. Adrenal inhibitors, and oils which relax the nervous system, include ylang-ylang and angelica root. Those which stimulate oestrogen include angelica, coriander, cypress and fennel. A correlation can be seen between the adrenal glands and the autonomic nervous system, in that both of them produce a substance called *noradrenaline*, which is, therefore, both an endocrine hormone and, in a different capacity, a neurochemical. Neurochemicals or transmitter chemicals are known to influence mood in various ways through their effect on the nerves in the brain.

While most essential oils possess very definite, individual healing properties there are times when an oil can do one of two things, according to the needs of the individual. Essential oils of *garlic* and *hyssop* both have a *normalizing* effect on blood pressure. If it is too high, using one of these oils will lead to a reduction in blood pressure. If it is too low, these oils will each increase it. Interestingly a study on the effect of hyssop oil on blood pressure found that it first went up, then down, then back to normal, almost as if the essential oil was testing out the pressure to see if it needed adjusting up or down.[22] Normalizing effects on the nervous system are quite common in essential oils. *Bergamot* or *geranium* oil, in particular, will either stimulate or sedate according to the needs of the individual. A recent Japanese study on the effects of essential oils on the central nervous system found that geranium oil stimulated some subjects and sedated others. This type of normalizing effect is not found in chemical drugs, and does not apply to all essential oils, but it can also be seen in a few herbal remedies. In *The Healing Arts*[11] Ted Kaptchuk and Michael Croucher state that: 'The action of Chinese angelica root on the uterus is unexplainable by the one-drug, one-effect theory; it can both relax a tight uterus and contract a loose one.' In so far as it does exist, the normalizing phenomenon demonstrates the versatility of natural remedies, and their appropriateness for helping with problems of 'natural balance'.

Dynamic Remedies

Essential oils are dynamic in more than one sense. They are highly sensitive organic liquids which, if not kept under the right conditions, will deteriorate. They will lose their healing potential, or we might say 'life force', and in this sense they are dynamic liquids. When applied to the body, they do act quite rapidly. They easily diffuse through the skin and into the body, and they can also penetrate through the walls of blood vessels and body tissues. They are dynamic because they go in, do their thing and then exit smartly from the body. In fact one reason for diluting them in vegetable oil is to slow them down a little. Although they do not remain in the body for more than three or four hours, they trigger off a healing process which may continue for days or even weeks after.

They are dynamic because they act on more than one level, influencing organs, functions, tissues, fluids, cells and subtle energy. They are also dynamic in the sense that high dilutions are sometimes effective. A study on the effect of lemon oil in stimulating the release of mucus on the lungs found that doses equivalent to an average person inhaling either sixty-eight drops or one-thirtieth of a drop were both effective. Doses in between were much less effective.

Essential oils are also dynamic because they are *synergistic*. Synergism means 'working together in harmony', and essential oils generally work better when mixed with other essential oils. Mixtures of between two and five oils are the norm in all branches of aromatherapy; for some reason using more than five or six oils seems to be counter-productive. Instead of an increased potency, you start to get a decrease. The fact of blending oils together is not sufficient in itself to ensure increased potency – much depends on which oils are blended and for what purpose. An eloquent example of synergism can be found in a study of the anti-bacterial effects of thirty-five essential oils carried out in 1958.[23] The authors first tested each of the oils against five disease-causing bacteria, and then tested the same oils in combinations of two, and then three. None of the dual blends showed any increased effect, but 20 per cent of the triple blends did. The most effective blend against these particular bacteria was eucalyptus, cinnamon and juniper, and it was 29 per cent more effective than would be expected from the individual effectiveness of the same oils.

The synergistic effect is also referred to by Valnet in his discussion of electrical resistance.[3] He gives an example of four essential oils: clove, thyme, lavender and peppermint. The electrical resistance of this mixture, which one would expect to be 3275, is in fact 17 000, a figure five times higher. The resistance of the mixture is much higher than that of its component essences. Aromatherapy blends do not always achieve synergism, but when they do, the result is considerably greater than the sum of its parts.

It is worth noting that the French aromatherapy doctors, working from the aromatogram (see next section), use mixtures of essential oils, rather than opting simply for the most effective oil. In holistic aromatherapy blends have always been used since the concept of the 'individual prescription' was introduced by Maury. Blends do have other advantages. A perfume is an example of a kind of synergism at work, since it aims to be 'a mixture in which the whole smells nicer than any of its ingredients'. In the same way simple blends of essential oils generally have a more appealing fragrance than single oils. Quite apart from its aesthetic value, this does lead to a greater degree of acceptance by the patient, which can be important when treating psychological or stress-related disorders. By using mixtures of oils it is possible to create a remedy which is finely tuned to the needs of the individual. From a selection of only twenty-five essential oils there are over 15000 possible blends of two, three or four essences.

Synergism also has another dimension. The properties of an essential oil can be influenced in different directions according to which oils it is mixed with. Bergamot oil is a good example. Blend it with jasmine, and it takes on an erogenic capacity; mix it with orange blossom, and its sedative action will predominate; in combination with lavender or tea-tree it becomes much more of an antiseptic; and mixing it with rosemary brings out its refreshing, stimulating nature. Bergamot is one of the most adaptable of all essential oils.

Protection/Prevention

There are a number of ways in which essential oils are either protective or preventive. Just as many of them perform a protective role in the plant,* they also protect us

* In many plants the evaporation of essential oil from the plant surface acts as a defence against damage by bacteria, fungi or pests.

Table 2. The effectiveness of a selection of essential oils against particular bacteria

Essential oil	Dilution	Bacterium	Related problem
Tea-tree[26]	1:200	Streptococcus	Throat infections
Sandalwood[27]	1:64 000	*Staph. aureus*	Infected wounds, Abscesses, boils
Thyme[25]	1:2000	*E. Coli*	Some kidney infections
Tea-tree[26]	1:12 800	Gonococcus	Gonorrhoea
Tea-tree[26]	1:200	Pneumococcus	Pneumonia
Lemon[25]	1:2000	*C. diphtheriae*	Diphtheria
Cinnamon[3]	1:300	Typhus bacillus	Typhus
Clove bud[3]	1:6000	*M. tuberculosis*	Tuberculosis

from bacteria, viruses, fungi, parasites, allergens and toxins. Since the first in 1887 there have been hundreds of laboratory tests which have demonstrated the effectiveness of essential oils against bacteria. All essential oils have anti-bacterial properties, but each oil is only effective against certain bacteria. At the same time as being toxic to bacteria, most of the oils are completely non-toxic to the human organism, the best example of this being tea-tree oil. It is the single most effective and least harmful anti-microbial essential oil (see Table 2). It is also effective against *Candida albicans*, the fungus which causes thrush, and against *Trichomonas vaginalis*, a tiny creature often responsible for vaginal infections.

In 1971 an Indian study was published which showed that lemongrass oil was slightly more effective against *Staph. aureus* than penicillin, and much more so than streptomycin.[24] *Staph. aureus* is one of the organisms most susceptible to essential oils, and it is usually rife in infected wounds. Valnet personally confirmed the conclusions of laboratory tests during the Second World War when, as an army surgeon, he used essential oils solutions as antiseptics in the treatment of battle wounds. In fact essential oils had been used for this same purpose as early as the seventeenth century. In his book *The Practice of Aromatherapy* Valnet cites the case of a thirty-one-year-old man whom he treated for pulmonary tuberculosis in 1958. A major operation had been recommended, but the patient refused this, and underwent an intense course of aromatherapy treatment instead. He was given daily nasal sprays, and aromatic enemas which proved successful, and twelve years later he was still in excellent health. On page 41 there is an example of garlic oil, another potent antiseptic, being used to treat TB in a US hospital. Many other cases could be listed of virtually every type of infectious disease being treated with aromatherapy. This has been pioneered by a number of French doctors, whose 'secret weapon' is called the *aromatogram*.[3]

The aromatogram is the holistic answer to treating infections. Very simply it involves taking a swab from an infected area of the patient, 'culturing' it in a laboratory (causing the bacteria to multiply rapidly) and then testing perhaps ten or fifteen different essences to find out which are the most effective. Three or four of these oils are then prescribed for the patient, usually to take orally as capsules. In this way the doctor can be sure that he is giving the most appropriate remedy for the individual patient. It is not even necessary to know exactly which bacteria are causing the infection. Not all French aromatherapy doctors ascribe to holistic principles, but virtually all of them swear by the aromatogram.

The culturing is performed in clear dishes, and one measured drop of each essential oil to be tested is placed on to the culture (Figure 5). After several hours there is a visible circle around each of the essence drops which has been able to kill off the bacteria. The diameter of this circle, which is known as the *zone of inhibition*, is then care-

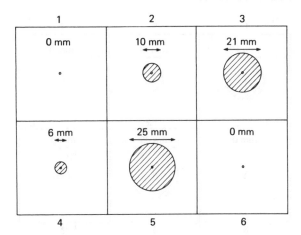

Figure 5. Hypothetical example of an aromatogram. Six different essential oils, here identified only by number, are being tested against one bacterial culture from the body of a patient. The shaded area is known as the 'area of inhibition' and shows how effective each oil is against the bacteria. In this case essential oils 3 and 5 would be used to treat the patient.

fully measured in millimetres. The larger it is, the more effective that essential oil has been against the cultured bacteria. If the oil is ineffective there will be no zone of inhibition.

An example of this process at work is given in *The Healing Arts*,[11] in which the authors describe a visit to the Parisian surgery of Dr Paul Belaiche. Belaiche was the first university professor of any kind of alternative medicine in Europe, and holds the chair of phytotherapy (plant therapy) at the Faculty of Medicine in the Université de Paris Nord. His treatment for a middle-aged woman suffering from a chronic urinary infection is described. She had endured years of unsuccessful conventional treatment, including antibiotics, the surgical stretching of her urethra and psychiatric help. Belaiche obtained a urine sample from the patient and asked her to return the following day. In the meantime, 'he tested the essential oils of seventy plants on cultures of the urine. The next day he prescribed various oils with anti-bacterial . . . properties; they were the oils that had reacted positively on the plates of urine culture. He prescribed with confidence. Dr Belaiche has achieved a success rate of better than 80 per cent with herbal treatment of several thousand women suffering from cystitis who had failed to respond to conventional treatment.'

A great many essential oils act against fungi, which cause common problems such as thrush, ringworm and athlete's foot. Viruses are surely the most insidious of all micro-organisms. Unlike bacteria they invade and take control of our own body cells, and so they are much more difficult for the immune system to identify and attack. Amongst the problems caused by viruses are colds, influenza, herpes (all types), chicken pox and measles. There are few substances, natural or synthetic, which are effective against viruses, but among them are certain essential oils. These include cinnamon, thyme, black pepper, eucalyptus, tea-tree (some influenza and cold viruses), lavender (herpes simplex, or cold sores; possibly also effective for genital herpes) and geranium (herpes zoster, or shingles).[3,28,29] Since there is hard evidence of the anti-viral effect of some of the oils, especially regarding influenza, there remains the remote possibility that aromatherapy may hold some kind of answer to the A I D S problem.

Essential oils have proved to be very effective against parasites, including lice, crabs, scabies, intestinal worms and trichomonas. While they are toxic to the parasites, essential oils are not toxic to the human organism. Benzyl benzoate, an aromatic chemical, is one of the few aromatic substances to enjoy official recognition. It is used as an external application in the treatment of scabies. Benzyl benzoate occurs naturally in oils of ylang-ylang, tuberose and hyacinth, but only in small quantities. The anti-parasitic action of essential oils has been recognized and used for the last 1000 years.

The anti-toxic action which many of the oils demonstrate may be seen in their effectiveness against the poison from insect bites and stings. Lavender and tea-tree are both effective against mosquito bites, and the sting of bee or wasp. Tea-tree has some effect on the poisonous bite of the funnel-web spider (see p. 195) and lavender is reputed to have a similar neutralizing effect on the bite of the black widow spider (see p. 175). These are the two most poisonous spiders known to man, and their bites are usually fatal. A number of essential oils appear to counteract the toxic effects of alcohol, notably rose. Oils of juniper and angelica root are believed to reduce excesses of *uric acid* in the blood, which usually occurs in gout and rheumatism. Other toxins, such as urea, and oxalic or lactic acids, are eliminated by certain essential oils. There is also reason to believe that aromatherapy can help with the problem of allergies. Many people with hay fever respond well to rose oil, and other allergic conditions, including food allergies, often yield to rose or yarrow.

In its preventive role aromatherapy also has an *indirect* answer to infection. The body's capacity to react to invasion (which is sometimes labelled *infection* and sometimes *allergy*) can be lowered by physical, mental or emotional exhaustion. The response to invasion is called the *immune response* and if it is completely knocked out the body is at the mercy of any invading organism. This is what sometimes happens to transplant patients, whose immune systems have to be lowered so that their bodies do not reject the new tissues. It is also what happens to people who contract A I D S. Some types of cancer are now thought to be related to a weakness in the immune system, and stimulation of it is being tried out as a form of cancer treatment. In his book *Maximum Immunity*[30] Michael A. Weiner comments: 'The age of antibiotics is fast coming to a close. Because of their great numbers, viruses and bacteria have quickly evolved resistant strains for almost every major man-made pharmaceutical. Positive, preventive health is becoming more and more important.' Not only do essential oils not have all the drawbacks associated with antibiotic drugs, they also help to stimulate the body's natural defence – the immune system. Many things are known to stimulate the immune system, including general well-being and happiness, improved nutrition, most types of massage and most essential oils. Essential oils will, I believe, largely take the place of antibiotics in years to come.

It has been demonstrated that rats which are frequently handled during infancy have a more competent immune system than rats which are not handled. Montagu[7] calls it a 'quite remarkable finding'. Naturopath Leon Chaitow apparently finds it less remarkable, saying, 'There is ample evidence of overall increase in immune function when relaxation is achieved via soft tissue massage.'

It has been said that all essential oils stimulate the formation of *phagocytes*, the white blood cells which gobble up invading bacteria. In a German book about the pharmaceutical effects of essential oils, published in 1906,[31] Rudolf Kobert spoke of essential oils stimulating the creation of anti-toxins, which he felt would eventually prove to be one of their most important functions. The ability of essential oils to stimulate the immune system is referred to by Rovesti, who says that this effect takes place whether the oils are applied by massage, inhalation or by mouth. He refers to a compatriot, Benedicenti, who 'foresaw preparations based on essences of bergamot, lavender and lemon to stimulate a "curative leucocytosis" in various types of infection'. Other essential oils have been referred to as leucocytosis stimulants.[31,32] In 1964 a study by H. M. Gattefossé (son of the man who coined the word aromatherapy) found that all essential oils stimulate *phagocytosis*, to varying degrees[33] (phagocytosis is the ability of white blood cells to gobble up invading bugs).

It is evident that both massage and essential oils, perhaps in different ways, are able to stimulate the body's natural defence systems. This, it should be said, is likely to have more effect in someone who is relaxed at the time of treatment. Here we have all the ingredients of an aromatherapy session – massage, essential oils and relaxation. Anyone who is 'run down' or prone to infections will benefit from the immuno-stimulating effects of aromatherapy.

Essential oils are quite good solvents. Whenever you spill some and wipe it up, it leaves the surface remarkably clean, and they will generally perform as well as pure alcohol for cleansing purposes. Most effective are lemon and grapefruit oils, which have also been shown to dissolve gall stones. This is due to their very high content (65–95 per cent) of terpenes, especially *limonene*. Valnet recommends oils of lemon, pine and terebinth for gall stones, all of which happen to have a very high terpene content. Peppermint, rosemary and bergamot, not so high in terpenes, have also been found useful. Oils of camomile, geranium, lemon and juniper have all been found of service in helping to dissolve or eliminate urinary stones. None of these essences have any dissolving or damaging effect on mucous membrane, or other normal body tissues.[34] According to the biologist P. V. Marchesseau essential oils in general 'cleanse the walls of blood vessels, the gall bladder, the kidneys and the articulations, contributing towards the dissolving of stones and facilitating their expulsion'.

Some essential oils act as blood cleansers/purifiers. These include angelica root and juniper, which, as we have already seen, promote the elimination of uric acid, and are useful in the treatment of gout and rheumatoid arthritis. High blood-urea levels, which occur in some kidney diseases, are reduced by camomile oil, and lactic acid, a waste product of muscular action, would appear to be eliminated by oils of lemongrass and rosemary, which are so effective in dealing with muscular aches. Marchesseau comments that essential oils 'increase the fluidity of blood and lymph, thereby helping to eliminate residues of a colloidal nature'. There is no hard evidence that I know of to the effect that essential oils prevent or dissolve deposits (mainly composed of cholesterol) on the walls of arteries (this problem, known as *atheroma* leads to arteriosclerosis, or hardening of the arteries, and sometimes to stroke or angina). However, Valnet recommends oils of garlic, lemon and juniper for the treatment of arteriosclerosis, and we are safe in assuming that some preventive or curative action is probable here.

The notion that garlic thins the blood now has scientific backing and is attributed to a newly identified substance named 'ajoene', a constituent of fresh garlic.[35] Trials are under way for the treatment of thrombosis and the prevention of clotting during surgery.

Many essential oils stimulate elimination through one route or another. Marchesseau points out that : 'They stimulate all the drainage ducts for the elimination of metabolic residues and of toxic products, the cutaneous glands, the lungs, kidneys and intestines, thus also acting as disintoxicants.' Among the most effect diuretic (urine-promoting) essences is juniper, which acts by enhancing the filtration action of the kidneys, and by increasing the amount of potassium, sodium and chlorine excreted.[36] Few essential oils act as laxatives, but one of the most expensive, rose oil, is effective here, and rosemary and marjoram are also of use. Other oils act as *expectorants*, stimulating the removal of heavy mucous in the lungs and bronchial tubes. This is helpful in virtually all respiratory conditions, and the most helpful oils include eucalyptus, tea-tree, lemon, lavender, peppermint and sandalwood. Other oils act on the skin, one of the body's major eliminative organs. These oils, known as *sudorifics*, include rosemary, hyssop and camomile, and they stimulate elimination through the sweat glands. Altogether, essential oils have a multiple effect in promoting cleansing and elimination in the body and in helping to keep it free from excesses of waste substances.

Aromatherapy is preventive in many ways, more than I can list here. We have already seen that it can stimulate the immune system (guarding against infection), prevent the build-up of toxic deposits in the body and counteract the damaging effects of stress. By these and similar preventive measures many forms of ill health are avoidable. Many of those who have aromatherapy treatments appreciate its preventive benefits. They will perhaps not undergo any dramatic cures, but they have found from experience that 'aromatherapy keeps the doctor away'.

Methods of application

In holistic aromatherapy the principal method of application is through the skin, by massaging in a mixture of essential and vegetable oils. Other means of application may be used as well as massage, but these are generally regarded as being supplementary methods. In clinical aromatherapy it is the other way around; applying oils by inhalation, by douche, suppository, or orally are the principal means of application, and massage usually does not figure at all. Essential oils can also be used in mouth-washes and gargles, in baths, compresses, enemas and even injections. Different methods may be suitable according to which part of the body the oils need to be delivered to. Inhalation, for example, is the best method of direct delivery to the lungs and sinuses, and also affects the nervous system through the sense of smell (see Chapter 5). Gargles would be used for throat infections, douches for vaginal problems and so on. Because of their volatile, solvent and antiseptic properties essential oil inhalations are especially effective in the treatment of sinus infections. I was told by an English doctor that they would also be invaluable for treating local infections. Applied to the skin the oils are able to penetrate directly to the site of infection. Not only are they better able to diffuse through body tissue than antibiotics, but they do not have to be taken by mouth and then find their way to the problem through the blood supply.

Taking essential oils by mouth is the normal method in France for dealing with infectious diseases. This has been the subject of some controversy in the UK, since some people feel that it could be more dangerous than rubbing diluted oils into the skin. In fact this is not so, but I feel the matter is somewhat academic, since holistic aromatherapy does not require that the oils be taken orally. Nevertheless, oral application is especially suitable for certain digestive problems and for urinary infections. If events follow a logical course then doctors and herbalists will gradually take to giving oral aromatherapy for certain infections and other problems, and holistic aromatherapists will stick to the other methods, principally massage. It is an interesting fact that oral application and whole-body massage deliver the same quantity of essential oil – about three drops – into the bloodstream. The various pathways followed by essential oils are shown in Figure 6.

Research

Modern aromatherapy benefits from a unique combination of research areas:

the medicinal properties of essential oils;
olfaction and the sense of smell;
the psychological effects of odours and essential oils;
the skin – its permeability and the importance of the sense of touch;
the therapeutic effects of both soft-tissue and pressure-point massage;
chemical, toxicological and other research on essential oils intended for the fragrance and flavour industries.

It is largely thanks to the fact that essential oils are so widely used by the fragrance and flavour industries that they have been investigated so thoroughly. Certainly most

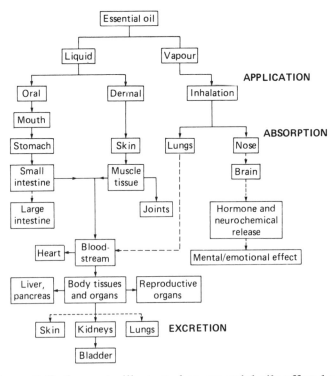

Figure 6. Pathways to illustrate how essential oils affect body and mind. (The dotted lines indicate either a nerve message or a very small amount of actual essential oil.)

of the studies referred to in this book were not carried out with aromatherapy in mind. However, complementary medicine is growing so rapidly that its research base desperately needs to do some catching up. A survey carried out by *Which?* magazine in 1986 revealed that, of those who had tried a form of complementary medicine, 82 per cent claimed to have been cured or improved, 74 per cent said that they would definitely go back for more, and 69 per cent said that they would recommend it to someone else with a similar complaint.

In the UK the Research Council for Complementary Medicine has been set up to encourage and help sponsor such research. The Association of Tisserand Aroma-therapists is currently involved in two projects concerning aromatherapy. A three-year study at Glasgow University has been set up to investigate the best ways to research complementary medicine. This is a very worthwhile venture, since natural medicines do not always work on a 'this remedy for that ailment' basis. Researching the clinical effects of essential oils is relatively simple. We might conclude, for instance, that 'tea-tree oil has a curative effect on 75 per cent of women with vaginal infections'. If prescribed for a group of 100 women it would therefore work for seventy-five of them, but not for the other twenty-five. In holistic medicine remedies are selected with many factors in mind, and quite different remedies may be given to patients with apparently the same problem. In the ideal situation the same 100 women would *all* be cured because dietary, psychological and subtle energy factors would all be taken into account, as would their individual responsiveness to essential oils. I do not pretend that the reality lives up to the ideal, at least not yet. However, new methods of research should lead to a deeper understanding of the complexities of holistic medicine.

A further complexity confronts aromatherapy research, since in its holistic form treatment consists of essential oils *plus massage*. A research study including both of these might easily conclude that the treatment is effective, but we would probably be no wiser as to *why* and *how* it works. How much is due to the essential oil, how much to the massage and how much to the presence of the therapist? At present we can only guess, and many of us are not really concerned anyway, as long as the treatment works. However, this would present an interesting and very challenging project. In the meantime we can say that aromatherapy has a sound basis of 'circumstantial evidence' already, and much groundwork has been achieved so far this century. What is needed now are clinical trials which, as far as possible, take the 'holistic factor' into account.

CHAPTER FOUR

ALL MANNER OF DISEASES

Quintessence they name to be, the chief and the heavenliest power or vertue in any plant ... which by ye force and puritie of the hoale substance ... conserveth the good health of mans body, prolongeth a mans youthe, differeth age, and putteth away all manner of diseases.

Conrad Gesner, 1559

Theories, laboratory experiments and clinical trials have all been referred to so far, but for many of us the real proof of any therapy is in how it performs in practice. I decided not to fill this chapter with evidence that 'rosemary oil stimulates respiration' or that 'lavender oil lowers blood pressure', but to fill it, instead, with case histories. To make it more interesting I have included cases from a number of different therapists, and have tried to cover a reasonable range of disorders. Since it treats the person, as much as the major complaint, holistic aromatherapy can help in many more conditions than are included in this chapter. In the majority of cases the essential oils used were successful because they suited the individual patient. The same oils may not be as effective in every similar case. The massage, dietary advice, and what we might call the 'therapist factor' also play a significant role in the healing process, and many of the cases illustrate the importance of the holistic approach. Others show that using the most appropriate essential oils is sometimes enough. A few are more anecdotes than case histories. Some I have commented on, and some I have not, but each one has its own, special story to tell.

I have included only cases which have a successful conclusion. Failures and semi-successes can be educational for aromatherapists, but are not appropriate here. However, I must counterbalance this deliberate omission by emphasizing that aromatherapy is by no means always successful. It has its share of failures as does any other form of medicine. (Success rates are not easy to evaluate, and I have no real figures to go on, but I would say that a competent aromatherapist can expect a success rate of between 70 and 85 per cent.) Each case is written in the words of the aromatherapist who gave the treatment, but I have done a little editing so that each one follows roughly the same pattern. The patients' names are sometimes real, and sometimes fictional, but the cases are all real, as are the therapists' names. The essential oils used are always mentioned, but the fact that they are used in dilution is not. For massage they are normally diluted to between 2 and 5 per cent.

Case Histories

Eczema (therapist: Christine Westwood)

Dawn, a twenty-five-year-old London publishing executive, had suffered from red, weeping eczema on both hands since early childhood. Eczema was diagnosed when she was about eighteen months old by the family general practitioner. Since that time she had used a number of medicinal creams, none of which had helped very much. The skin of her hands itched intensely, and was often a mess of small open sores. Her doctor could only suggest: 'Keep using the cream and don't worry.' Dawn also suffered from occasional migraines, aggravated by the stress of work, and had had periods of insomnia since the death of a close friend. Two minor problems were constipation and poor circulation.

At first I saw her weekly, and later monthly. I massaged

her back, stomach, face and feet with a blend of juniper, frankincense and camomile.* I felt that the frankincense in particular would help her to relax, and to overcome her fears around sleeping. I also made up an ointment for her to use at home with juniper, frankincense and lavender to heal the skin. After her first visit Dawn said that she was sleeping much better, and during the next few visits her constipation and poor circulation both improved and her eczema started to clear. After further treatments it became apparent that her migraines had relented and the eczema continued to improve. During this time Dawn became noticeably more cheerful and confident in herself. I also gave her various vitamin and mineral supplements to support and strengthen her system during the period of treatment, which lasted for six months. One year later Dawn's hands are still completely clear, although if she eats chocolate it usually causes a little redness for a couple of days.

Dawn herself made the following comments, reported in a national newspaper in May 1986: 'I was sceptical about aromatherapy, but would have tried anything. It has changed my life. My hands are almost better, I no longer have the terrible itching, and I'm sleeping better than I ever thought possible.'

Psoriasis (therapist: Valerie Worwood)

Mrs N. had infantile eczema which gradually developed into psoriasis, diagnosed by her doctor when she was in her late thirties. A fifty-year-old housewife, she had been married twice. She told me that she had been unhappy as a child, and other children had always been very unkind to

---

* In this, and the other cases in which 'camomile' is mentioned, it refers to Roman camomile, unless otherwise stated.

her because of her skin condition. Her first husband had a violent temper, and her condition had worsened since the time of her first marriage. When she first came to see me she was in such a bad state that at first I decided I would not treat her. The psoriasis literally covered her from head to toe, and she never wore skirts because of her legs and always wore thick tights and a headscarf. It may sound corny, but she begged me, with tears in her eyes, to at least try to help her.

She had already been to a hypnotherapist, a herbalist and a homoeopathic doctor and other therapists. She had used creams of various descriptions, had undergone every test in the book, and some of the other therapies she tried seemed to make the condition worse. She did have a nervous disposition and her skin was splitting and bleeding in parts; the prospects were not good, and any kind of body massage was quite out of the question. Bathing and compresses seemed the best answer, and when she came for treatment I applied compresses over her whole body for ten minutes at a time. First a compress of camomile and lavender, then one also with bergamot, and finally one with the previous three oils plus geranium. After the very first compress a slight improvement was noticeable, and by the time I removed the third her waist was becoming white instead of red. It was actually changing before my eyes. I had never experienced this before, and was a little unsure of what was happening. We started the cycle again, and I sent her home with a bottle of oil to use in her bath. It contained the third compress formula, and she was instructed not to use it directly on her body.

She returned three days later in tears. Her hands had cleared, and her face was also clear, except for a small crusty area around the hair-line. Two weeks later her whole body had cleared, except for the stubborn hair-line area, which took a further month to clear. She came for weekly treatments for three months, and then once every three months for two years. She now remains clear of psoriasis and of eczema, and is convinced that if aromatherapy had been known to her at an early age she would have avoided a lifetime of misery. After a few weeks of treatment I did suggest some changes in her diet, and she cut down on red meat, cut out dairy products and ate more fresh vegetables.

COMMENT

Why aromatherapy should work in this case, and so dramatically, when hypnotherapy, herbal and homoeopathic medicine had all failed to produce results I do not know. All of these have been successful in other cases of psoriasis. For reasons as yet little understood, some people respond better to one therapy than to another. This case is also interesting because it is very clear that neither faith nor massage played any part, certainly in the initial stages.

Acne rosacea (therapist: Robert Gibson*)

Acne rosacea should not be confused with common acne, since it is a quite different condition. It is characterized by excessive redness on the cheeks and nose (which cannot be seen in a black-and-white photograph) and by greasiness, enlarged pores and lumpy swellings, the skin becomes thick, and is often permanently scarred. The psychological impact on the patient can lead to social withdrawal and severe depression.

The patient, Irene, consulted a dermatologist when she developed small spots on her face and neck in her late

---

* Mr Gibson, a member of the Institute of Trichologists in Glasgow, practises many therapies, including aromatherapy.

twenties. Until then her skin had been admired for its clarity, tone and freshness. She was prescribed panoxyl gel for external use and oxytetracycline to be taken orally. This treatment was continued without pause for five years, during which time her condition got progressively worse. The panoxyl gel caused painful fissures around the mouth, and her face and neck became covered in abscesses and cysts. These were up to one inch in diameter, and half-an-inch deep, discharging blood-stained fluid and pus. At this point in time the patient was given a medical certificate by her general practitioner with the express advice to go and hide for a month.

She then decided to forsake conventional treatment, and was admitted to a homoeopathic hospital as an in-patient for five weeks. Blood tests revealed that staphylococci were 'running riot' and that many of the white blood cells were 'breaking up' due to toxins released by the bacteria. On being discharged from the hospital she consulted me about her condition. With the approval of one of the homoeopathic doctors I started treating her once a week. After five weeks she went to the Glasgow Western Infirmary for a skin biopsy, arranged by the homoeopathic doctor. The biopsy should have taken no more than one hour, but she was kept as an in-patient for a month by the Professor of Dermatology, who wished to re-establish oxytetracycline therapy. This was refused by the patient, so a substitute treatment was given involving the application of sulphur and zinc paste and then injections into the largest cysts. This temporarily reduced the degree of suppuration, but the redness and irritation became worse. As soon as this therapy ceased, the suppuration swiftly returned, as bad as ever. Dermatologists mocked the idea of alternative or aromatherapy treatment, saying that *nothing* would reduce the inflammation, never mind remove it, and that only medical doctors had the necessary expertise to treat her condition.

After her discharge Irene did not consult me again for eighteen months. Finally she telephoned me from the Glasgow Royal Infirmary, where she was about to undergo yet another type of treatment. I reminded her that I was convinced I could help her, and that she had nothing to lose, as aromatherapy would not harm her. Unfortunately treatment had to be deferred for a while since I was undergoing treatment for a lymphatic tumour. Finally we recommenced aromatherapy treatment.

I gave Irene some dietary advice and suggested specific vitamin and mineral supplements to her. Through unavoidable circumstances she was not able to follow this advice, and consequently nutrition played no part in her recovery. Nor was I able to use hypnotherapy and relaxation due to my own low state and need for therapy at the time. The success of the treatment was due completely to facial massage and the aromatic products applied to the skin. An important facet of the massage was *lymphatic drainage*, which helps to eliminate the toxins released by the other movements. A number of essential oils played a part in the treatment, the main ones being as follows:

To calm and oxidize: mint and bitter orange;
To detoxify: linden blossom, rosemary, wild camomile;
To improve tone of facial muscles and capillary walls: mint, bay laurel, rosemary;
As a decongestive: linden blossom, bitter orange, bay laurel.

In the beginning we tried to bring to a head as many of the large pustules as possible. After a slight initial worsening the condition improved steadily over the first few weeks, and eventually cleared from the forehead downwards, with the neck being the last area to clear. (The scalp also required treatment, and without this the face might well have become reinfected.) After three months of treatment I decided to take some photographs, although by this time the condition was much improved, and the upper part of the face had begun to clear [see Figure 7(a)].

I saw Irene every week for eight months, and she then continued with home treatments, which she had been doing since the beginning, for a further four months. After one year of treatment the appearance of her skin had improved to an astonishing degree [Figure 7(b)]. The pustules and lumps had disappeared, and the skin had become soft and pliable once more. Make-up, which used to literally slide off after two hours, now remained stable, since the greasiness had

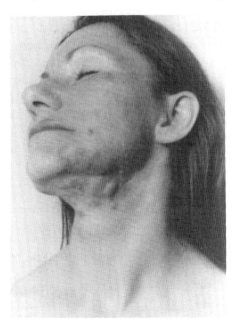

Figure 7. (a) After three months. The pustular swellings are still visible on the lower face and neck. The red inflammation, still present at this time, does not show up in black and white.

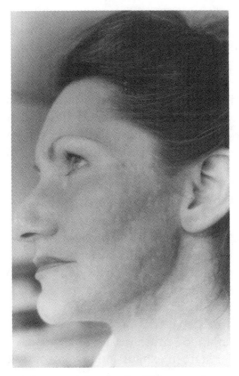

Figure 7. (b) After twelve months. The pustular swellings have gone completely, as has the inflammation. (Photograph courtesy of Robert Gibson)

almost completely gone. Most remarkably the characteristic inflammation on nose and cheeks had also gone, in spite of the claim by dermatologists that it could not be done. The ice-pick scarring had reduced, but was still noticeable. The tragedy is that the scarring, and five years of physical and psychological misery, could have been avoided had the condition been treated with aromatherapy from an early stage.

It is now more than four years since her last treatment, and Irene's skin has not only maintained its condition, but is continuing to improve. As a result of her experiences she has since undertaken several studies in the field of complementary medicine.

COMMENT

This case history shows that conventional treatment can be ineffective, suppressive, and can be harmful in the long term. Aromatherapy can take months or even years in very chronic cases, but in the end it heals by working *with* the body, not against it.

Verrucae (therapist: Patricia Davis)

Aged twenty-six years and five months pregnant at the time of her first visit, Kate had twenty-seven verrucae – twenty-one on her left foot and six on her right. Her medical history revealed that she had had glandular fever several times, and she currently had little resistance to infection and was lacking in physical energy. This had been a problem long before her recent pregnancy. Kate had problems holding down a job, either because of extensive sick-leave or because her state of exhaustion made working efficiently very difficult.

The verrucae had been treated conventionally for the past two years by cutting out and burning. It was clear that this problem was a result of a low level of immune response and so treatment was aimed at improving this. In addition, lemon oil was applied directly to the verrucae. Kate was given massage at weekly intervals to improve the function of her lymphatic system, and she applied the lemon oil to her feet at home. At the first session oils of geranium and rosemary were used. Although the idea was basically to stimulate she reported later that when she got home she slept for thirty-six hours, waking only to visit the toilet and drink a little water. When she finally woke up properly she felt more energetic than at any time in the past ten years, on her own reckoning.

At her third visit Kate reported a marked decrease in the number of verrucae on her left foot, with about eight of the smaller ones completely gone. There was no change on the right foot. This pattern of treatment continued almost to the end of her pregnancy. The verrucae would appear to be unchanged for a week or two, and then diminish very quickly. It eventually became clear that these periods followed the use of rosemary and geranium – I had been trying other oils during some of her visits. Kate also reported greatly increased levels of energy throughout this period.

Some four months later, shortly before the birth of Kate's baby, she had only six small verrucae on her left foot, and none on her right. She had not had a single cold, or any other infection, throughout the period of treatment, and she felt so well and energetic that she held a party for fifty people shortly before her expected confinement.

COMMENT
This case illustrates very well the importance of the holistic approach. Even for something as physical as verrucae, it was by treating the *patient*, and her immune system, that success was achieved.

Cellulitis (therapist: Patricia Davis)
Margaret was twenty-nine years old and a music teacher with a lot of responsibility in a girls' public school. She had heavy cellulitis on her thighs, hips and buttocks and a tendency to put on weight due to fluid retention. This became worse in hot weather, when her ankles would swell with

fluid. She had a noticeably pear-shaped figure. Her diet was very good, but she took no exercise and spent long periods either sitting at the piano or standing in class at school. She experienced quite a lot of anxiety in her job, including some friction with the head teacher.

Margaret had three weeks free from school during the Easter break, and had determined to 'do something' about her cellulitis in that time. She came to see me twice a week and I massaged the problem areas with essential oils of rosemary, fennel and geranium. She was very keen to do her bit, and carried out a gentle exercise and relaxation routine every day. She also went on a short fruit fast at the beginning of the holiday and made a few improvements in her diet. She also used a bath oil at home with juniper, lavender, geranium, bergamot and camomile. This was aimed at detoxifying and also at helping with her anxiety and occasional depression.

Results were immediately noticed. Margaret lost a lot of fluid, and her hip measurement reduced so fast that all her skirts were too big for her after ten days. As I was satisfied that the lymphatic system was now functioning much more efficiently, I incorporated a vigorous massage of the cellulitic areas in each treatment. She also used a proprietary massage glove in her daily bath as a back-up treatment. By the end of the three weeks there remained only one small, stubborn patch of cellulitis, about four inches square, in area, on the back of one thigh. I was puzzled by this, and asked if there was anything she did with one leg that she did not do with the other. After a moment's thought she replied: 'Yes, pedals!' She demonstrated her sitting position at the piano, which meant that the edge of the piano stool cut across one thigh, causing pressure just below the affected area.

As she was not able to continue with treatment on such an intensive basis once school had restarted, I gave her a supply of massage cream which I made up for her, with careful instructions on how to work on her own legs until they were entirely free of cellulitis.

COMMENT
This case history demonstrates that a patient's co-operation and involvement in their own healing process can often bring quicker results.

Fracture
This account, of a healthy thirteen-year-old-boy who broke a bone in one hand, is told by his mother, Susan Murdoch, an aromatherapist.

Jamie broke the little finger of his right hand near the knuckle joint while playing football in the summer of 1986. My husband, David, took him to casualty at Mount Vernon Hospital, Rickmansworth. Jamie's hand was very swollen and painful and, after X-rays, the doctor strapped it up saying that such a fracture would take some six weeks to heal.

Remembering that ginger oil was supposed to be very good for healing bones I decided to mix up an oil for Jamie's finger, hoping of course that it would speed up and improve the healing process. The recipe I used contained ginger oil, rosemary oil, juniper oil and lavender oil. Jamie rubbed the oil on his hand twice a day and also practised keeping the other joints mobile.

Three weeks later David took Jamie up to the Hand Clinic in Mount Vernon to see a Dr Smith. Unfortunately I was unable to go, but Jamie told me that evening: 'Mum, the doctor was totally amazed, he said the fracture had healed in half the time, and couldn't get over the fact that my hand didn't hurt when I moved it, or when the doctor asked me to clench my fist, or pulled my finger.' David and I were totally amazed as well, and I later wrote to Dr Smith, telling him about the oil, and saying that I would welcome any comments he had to make, but he did not reply.

COMMENT
This account is especially interesting, because the whole affair was, quite unwittingly, monitored by two hospital doctors. If the fracture had healed in four or five weeks, perhaps it would not be so impressive, but to heal completely in three weeks, half the normal time, is surely significant. It would not be surprising if aromatherapy can speed up the healing of bones, since we have already discussed the cell-stimulating effect of essential oils in relation to skin cells and white blood cells. If aromatherapy can speed up the healing of wounds, ulcers and burns, then why not broken bones as well?

Sprained ankle (therapist: Geraldine Howard)
Mary, a woman in her forties, was told by her doctor that she had a pulled tendon. She had the usual ankle-sprain symptoms of pain, bruising and swelling and was advised to rest her foot, using it as little as possible until the swelling reduced. After three days it had not improved and she sought my help. I made up an oil with rosemary, juniper and lavender for her to massage gently around the joint.

A little while after the first application of oil the swelling had reduced considerably. The bruising, which had been severe, also seemed to disappear very quickly, and after seven days the ankle was so much better that we were able to massage it. This, combined with regular applications of the oil, improved mobility and reduced pain to such a degree that it surprised even her doctor.

Arthritis (therapist: Christine Westwood)

Marion is a clerk typist in her late fifties. She experienced immobility and pain from arthritis, which had started several years ago in her shoulders. This was diagnosed in September 1985 at a private hospital in North London. Despite receiving regular physiotherapy, ultrasonic and hot-wax treatments at the hospital, her elbows and hands subsequently became affected. A number of X-rays were taken, which showed wear and tear in the joints.

I chose camomile for its soothing effect, and rosemary to stimulate the circulation and to aid the lymph system in releasing stored toxins around the affected joints. Lavender was also included to ease the pain and to facilitate deep relaxation. After her first visit she initially felt a little stiffer. This can often happen as the body relaxes and releases toxins into the system. After her second visit she commented that her arms were more mobile than they had been for years, and after this point she experienced no more stiffness at all.

When she came for her third treatment Marion told me that she had been troubled with backache during the last few days. On further enquiry it transpired that her arms had felt so much better that she had enthusiastically embarked on some gardening – something she had been unable to do for the last couple of years. The backache was soon remedied. During her weekly sessions, over a period of two months, she was also using a mixture of essential oils at home, to rub into the affected joints. It is now ten months since her first visit, and she remains free from symptoms. She now comes monthly for preventative health care because she feels that it helps her.

Spondylitis (therapist: Christine Westwood)

Carol was a little sceptical when she first came to see me, although she was willing to try anything. She had previously received osteopathy, homoeopathy and acupuncture, all to no avail. X-rays revealed that the fifth and sixth thoracic vertebrae (in between the shoulder blades) were slightly out of place and showed signs of arthritis. She was diagnosed by a homoeopathic doctor as having spondylitis – inflammation of the vertebrae. This was eight years ago, when Carol was forty. She suffered from constant tiredness and her back ached all over, but especially in her neck and lower back, even though the spondylitis was elsewhere. Her back also ached between the shoulder blades in the evening, when she sat down for any length of time, and she found it difficult to sit for the consultation. She was unable to do any housework, and every so often had to lie down on the floor to rest, since this afforded some relief from the pain. Her periods were also severe, and she usually spent the first day in bed.

Juniper, rosemary and lavender were the principal oils used. Treatment was given to ease the tension connected with the constant pain and to soothe the inflammation. Carol came for an initial treatment, then after two weeks and subsequently monthly. After the first treatment the pain had eased considerably and she felt much better in herself. On her third visit she said that she was delighted with her progress. Her back was much better, the spine felt freer and when she did feel some pain it did not last for long. She spent less time resting on her back. Her periods were also much less severe, and instead of resting in bed the last time she had played a round of golf.

Carol had a scar on her back from a boil which had been lanced thirty-three years previously. Amazingly the scar tissue healed completely after further back massages. I also gave her oils of juniper and lavender to use several times a week in the bath, which she found very beneficial. On her second visit I gave her some nutritional advice which she immediately took action on. She started to eat more fresh fruits and vegetables and to drink herb teas, and has since decided to become vegetarian. It is now seven months since she first came to see me, and she still comes once every month.

Sinusitis (therapist: Valerie Worwood)

When he came to see me Mr A. was in his late thirties and worked in a high-pressure advertising job which involved a great deal of travelling. The travel was his excuse for a terrible diet, and his work certainly contributed to his anxiety and extreme headaches. His sinus cavities were infected and congested, with pain and tenderness of the area around his nose.

Treatment was aimed at reducing the sinus congestion and inflammation, and also to clear his digestive system and his lungs of some mucous congestion. He came to me for weekly aromatherapy sessions, in which I used oils of rosemary, juniper, bergamot and hyssop.

He gave himself daily inhalations with lavender, tea-tree, eucalyptus and rosemary, and used cajuput, niaouli and lemon oils in his bath. He had no known food allergies, but he cut out dairy products and reduced his consumption of red meat and wheat products. A steady improvement took place during the first three weeks, after which his voice was noticeably clearer and deeper. Weekly treatments continued for a further three weeks, after which time his sinusitis had gone and his breathing was greatly improved. He is also much calmer, and his bowels are now functioning normally. He now comes to see me occasionally, as he puts it, 'to keep me in shape'.

Chronic bronchitis (therapist: Valerie Worwood)

This patient, a sixty-eight-year-old retired Ford worker, had been screened for TB by her doctor and was sent to me by a chiropractor who thought I could help. She had high blood pressure, infected tonsils and had smoked for the last fifty years. She also had a back problem, which was being attended to by her chiropractor. For years she had had a chronic, mucousy cough which never let up and left her completely exhausted. The mucus was occasionally streaked with blood and she was constantly breathless.

She was not prepared to consider cutting down, far less giving up, smoking. (I also suspected that she had a drinking problem, but this was never confirmed.) However, we did manage to agree on a sensible, wholefood diet, which she more or less stuck to the whole time. I decided to treat her with every possible means of application, including compresses (chamomile and lemon), body oils (cedarwood, cajuput, niaouli and hyssop), an oral prescription and inhalations (chamomile, lemon and thyme). I saw her once a week, and she also used oils daily at home.

During the first three weeks of treatment her condition worsened. Her cough became even more intense, and she became extremely tired and slept a great deal. After this point her cough eased considerably, her breathlessness disappeared and her energy level steadily increased. Soon she no longer felt tired, and was only coughing once a day on rising. After six months of treatment there is now no trace of bronchitis, and she seems perfectly fit and healthy. Her blood pressure has returned to normal and she has a very positive outlook on life.

COMMENT

A considerable reduction in smoking is usually essential for any real success in such cases. The first three weeks of treatment must have been quite a battle for both therapist and patient. In spite of the apparent deterioration in the condition they both stuck at it, and I would venture to suggest that determination had as much to do with the ultimate success as did the essential oils used.

Cardiac failure (therapist: Valerie Worwood)

I saw this lady in 1985, a sixty-five-year-old widowed restaurant proprietor. She had been active all her life, had three children, but had experienced more stress in her life than at any other time after the death of her husband, years before. She had an acute sense of loss and loneliness, her business gradually declined and soon after selling it she fell prey to cardiac failure. She had swollen legs due to excess fluid (dropsy), a high pulse rate and shortness of breath and palpitations on exertion.

I put her on a wholefood diet, with no tea, coffee or dairy produce. Treatment consisted of two short aromatherapy massage sessions (thirty minutes) per week for one month. The following month she came just once a week and she was then weaned on to one session per month. We used oils of geranium, cypress, hyssop and juniper for her physical condition, plus rose *otto* for her psychological state. During the second month bergamot oil was also added. This treatment continued for twelve months.

An improvement was seen after the first session. She felt much better psychologically, since she had found someone to help her, and use of the same oils at home enhanced her treatment. After the first few weeks her legs reduced, and she was able to see her ankles for the first time in years. After two months she suddenly realized that she was not getting short of breath any longer, and her blood pressure had returned to normal after the first month.

She now lives a normal life, has taken up tennis and

ballroom dancing and travels around Europe on coach trips. The condition of her legs and heart had previously prevented her from doing any of these. She now plans to re-marry.

COMMENT
This case shows the 'rejuvenating' effects of aromatherapy. Regardless of age, there is always hope, and aromatherapy can make it possible to return to living a healthy, active life.

Varicose veins and ulcers (therapist: Valerie Worwood)
This lady worked as a secretary and had varicose veins diagnosed when she was twelve years old. She had no treatment, although surgical removal of the veins was recommended when she was in her late teens. She declined, and her condition slowly worsened until she came to see me at age twenty-eight years. Her symptoms included heaviness in the legs, continued tiredness and intense itching (diagnosed by her general practitioner as 'itchy leg'). Betnovate cream was prescribed, but her condition worsened, leading to scaly patches (eczema) all over her legs with areas of blistering and ulcers with pus. No other treatment had been offered.

When I saw her she was in a highly emotional state, was severely depressed and would wear trousers instead of skirts as she was acutely embarrassed by the appearance of her legs. The ulcers had eaten deep into the flesh and there were signs of further ulcerated areas developing. I offered some nutritional advice, plus a suggestion to cut down on her smoking, which was aggravating a bronchial condition. I decided to massage her back and abdomen, using oils of cypress, geranium, clary sage and lavender. I also applied a steam-heated compress to her legs, with oils of geranium, cypress, lavender, tea-tree, yarrow and camomile. I saw her weekly for two weeks, and then monthly, and she applied compresses twice per day at home using the same blend of oils.

After two days the ulceration began to heal and the intense itching on the rest of her legs began to decrease. One week later the ulcers were practically gone and there remained only a pink-red scaly patch which gradually transformed into normal skin. Treatment was continued as before, and the eczema on the rest of her legs gradually cleared and has not returned. We continued treatment for twelve months, during which time the varicose condition lessened and her symptoms of tiredness, etc. went away. Subsequently I have been able to treat her bronchial problem and, with some persuasion, she finally gave up smoking.

Period pains (therapist: Valerie Worwood)

Miss C., aged twenty-eight years, suffered severe period pains which had been diagnosed by a medical practitioner as *spasmodic dysmenorrhoea*. With the onset of menstruation pain radiated from her back around the pelvic area. Each cycle seemed to get progressively worse, with constipation occurring a week prior to her period. This only aggravated the condition. She had tried all the usual treatments, including acupuncture, and was taking large doses of aspirin. She works as a secretary in the Civil Service, in quite a high position for someone of her age, and she has to work odd hours. This plays havoc with her diet, which is appalling – mainly junk food and large quantities of red meat, with hardly any fruit or vegetables. She was very keen to find help for her problem, as she feared it might eventually interfere with her chances of promotion at work.

Treatment started on the third day after menstruation

began, and consisted of whole-body massage with essential oils of rose, lavender, geranium, basil, cypress and fennel. This was changed after the second menstrual period. She attended for monthly treatments, and after four months the pain had diminished considerably and she was much fitter. She had more energy generally and was enjoying life more. She followed my advice regarding her diet, and now eats less red meat and more fruit, vegetables and raw salads. She is also doing more exercise, swimming and jogging, and is happy with her new life-style.

Her periods now last for only three days, with no premenstrual symptoms and very little pain. If she has been working overtime for a long while she soaks in a bath with the blend of oils I make up for her, and books in for a session, as she says, 'to put me back together again'.

Vaginal discharge (therapist: Valerie Worwood)

The patient had been troubled with this problem for several years, although a precise diagnosis was never forthcoming, other than 'inflammation of the uterus'. She had a continual, profuse discharge which resulted in extreme discomfort. Antibiotic and anti-inflammatory drugs had been prescribed but the condition persisted. Different antibiotic drugs were prescribed several times, but each time the condition cleared for a few days and then returned. She became very irritable and stressed by the vicious circle which she was living through, and because of the lack of an exact diagnosis.

I suggested that we try only relaxing treatments to enable the body to rebalance. She agreed and came for three weekly treatments. I gave her a general body massage concentrating on the abdomen and lower back; the oils used were rose, bergamot, camomile and sandalwood. After this time she was very much less stressed and continued to use the formula in her bath at home. However, the condition persisted and was not really any better. She was very keen for me to try an alternative to the antibiotics as her last course had finished. I decided on a combination of lavender, yarrow and sandalwood, which was used in a warm-water douche for a period of three days. She then inserted a tampon soaked in vegetable oil and lavender and repeated this for the next four days. After this time the pain and discharge had cleared up, and has not returned since.

COMMENT
It is interesting to compare the successful method of treatment described in these last two sentences with the treatment of both vaginitis and thrush with tea-tree oil, described on pages 192–3.

Thrush (therapist: Geraldine Howard)
When I saw Gillian she was in her thirties and was plagued by constantly recurring attacks of thrush. She had tried using the pessaries prescribed by her doctor, but had given them up since ultimately they did not help her at all. I suggested that she buy a douche, and use it with oils of bergamot, rose and lavender in the water. She welcomed my advice, and used the douche once a day at the onset of her next attack. After only two days the irritation was very much better, which was a great relief to her as the condition normally got worse over the first few days of an attack.

Within one week she was completely symptom-free and altogether suffered far less discomfort than normal. She continued with a weekly douche for several further weeks. One year later she had had only one mild attack, and she still uses the douche once a month just as a precaution. I have found that many people with less severe attacks respond well to a sitz bath with about ten drops of essential oil in the water. This usually clears an attack within a few days, although it is best to continue treatment for a little while.

COMMENT
This is one of the conditions which invariably responds well to aromatherapy (see p. 193 for more information about thrush, and details of a clinical trial on thrush patients using tea-tree oil).

Menopausal problems (therapist: Valerie Worwood)

This lady was fifty years old when she came to see me with menopausal problems. She was surprised to be having such problems, as her mother and grandmother had had an easy time through theirs. She had most of the problems associated with the menopause: night-sweats, tremors, extreme dryness of the vagina and terrible mood swings. Her family were very concerned about her changing moods (she was very happy in her marriage, and had a close, caring family). The night-sweats got progressively worse, and cold day-sweats now caused her acute embarrassment. She was quite distressed by the attitude of her general practitioner (a woman) who told her that it was something she would just have to put up with.

I suggested fortnightly visits, and hoped to alleviate her anxiety as well as the actual symptoms. I gave her a whole-body massage, and used essential oils of clary sage, geranium, fennel and violet leaf. This had a balancing effect which enabled the body to carry on with its hormonal change with much less disturbance and discomfort. The night-sweats began to diminish, and after six treatments her tension and mood swings had balanced out. Her vaginal secretions also increased, helped by the fennel oil, and she is now a very much happier woman. She now uses blended oils at home, and visits me once every two months for the relaxation benefit and for the refuge of knowing someone cares.

Personal anecdote

To round off this chapter I would like to include an account of an interesting event that happened while I was working in a Brighton Clinic.

A patient came into the clinic to see the acupuncturist, Marek Urbanowitcz. She was in her thirties, and had very bad earache in her right ear. She had come as an emergency, and had to wait until Marek had a few minutes to spare. As she sat in the waiting room the pain of her earache worsened, and the clinic receptionist showed her into an empty treatment room so she could lie down on the couch. I was free at the time, and went in really just to comfort her. She was lying on her left side, holding her head in her hands, almost desperate from the pain. She could hardly move or speak, and tears ran down her face. I recalled my own experience of earache as a child, and the almost un-bearable pain of it.

I went off to make up an oil for her, with that feeling (rare for an alternative therapist) of someone centre-stage in a desperate situation. I had to do something for her! As fate would have it, the previous evening I had been reading an article about aromatherapy treatment for ear infections. Suddenly remembering this added to my state of inspired fervour. I mixed up an oil with rosemary, lavender and tea-tree and, as gently as I could, rubbed it around the ear. The degree of the swelling was alarming. I also put a tiny wad of cotton wool in her ear, with neat essential oil on it. I stayed with her for ten or fifteen minutes holding my hands over the ear and switching my psyche into its 'healing mode. Then Marek arrived. He placed one needle near the centre of the swelling, one in her foot, and one somewhere else. I wrapped her in a blanket and left her to rest.

About fifty minutes later I heard a voice saying: 'Thank you very much, goodbye, I'm off now!' I was absolutely stunned, and could not believe it was the same person. She was almost completely back to normal – smiling, and full of life. I have never seen such a rapid recovery from anything, either before or since.

This is one of those cases where you do not know who or what should take the credit. Was it the oils, the acupuncture or the healing? Most likely it was the combination of the three which resulted in such a dramatic recovery. Certainly the patient cannot take the credit here, except for her bravery.

CHAPTER FIVE

THE PSYCHE

Of all the senses, none surely is so mysterious as that of smell . . . its effects upon the psyche are both wide and deep, at once obvious and subtle.

Daniel MacKenzie

Odiferous matter reaches regions of the brain which are not under conscious control; its perception affects our psychic life and transforms our predispositions.

Marguerite Maury

We have already discussed how essential oils in liquid form affect the physical body, but what about the aroma in aromatherapy? Is it really possible for the fragrance of an essential oil to influence our mood, our feelings, our state of mind, even our behaviour?

The compelling power of odours on the psyche has been recognized since the very earliest times. Aromatic woods, gums and herbs were burned to drive out 'evil spirits' and kyphi, an ancient Egyptian perfume, was said to 'lull to sleep, allay anxieties and brighten dreams'. In ancient Greece aromatic oils were often employed for their soporific, antidepressant or aphrodisiac properties, and it was recognized that certain odours could improve mental alertness and aid concentration.

The smoke from burning bay leaves was inhaled by the Oracle at Delphi to induce a trance-like state enabling communication with the gods. Dwight Hines (1977) (Ph.D. in Psychology, University of Maine) explains that odours are capable of creating: 'an emotional, ecstatic state of

consciousness that would render individuals more susceptible to religious experience',[1] and another author (1955)
has commented on the importance of perfumes in magic
rituals, religious ceremonies and nervous diseases, describing them as: 'modifiers of the spirit and of the senses'. In
1875 the use of odorants was suggested in the treatment of
the mentally ill, since it had been observed that the emotional effects of odours were very powerful. This was also
noted by Montaigne, who wrote: 'Physicians might draw
more use and good from odours than they do. For I have
often perceived, that according to their strength and quali-
tie, they change, and alter, and move my spirit, and work
strange effects in me.' More recently (1960), it has been
said that perfumes and aromas are: 'an important means
. . . of obtaining a change in psychic state . . . both by inspiration and by absorption through the skin'.

In ancient Egypt incense, perfumes, healing and magic
were all very closely related and very much a part of
everyday life. Although they have long since become
diversified, as have 'science' and 'mysticism', there seems
to be a healthy trend towards a new unity of thought. Just
as conventional and complementary medicine are now
slowly coming together, there are confident predictions that
the perfumery industry is moving towards 'therapeutic
perfumes'. While the content of these may be more synthetic
than natural, there is also the hope that the link with aromatherapy will lead to a wider use of natural ingredients.

Fragrance researchers are discovering that odours can
and do influence mood, evoke emotions, counteract stress
and reduce high blood pressure.[2] As an aromatherapist I
have witnessed many times how aromatherapy makes
people feel better in themselves, improving temperament,
aiding relaxation and consequently increasing confidence,
energy levels and the ability to cope with stress. To explain

how essential oils can affect us in this way we must first explore the various connections between the sense of smell and the brain, or nervous system.

Babies born with *anencephaly*, a rare and lethal defect in which the brain fails to develop, are also born without a nose, although the other sense organs are intact. In evolutionary terms the first senses to develop are those of touch and smell. Experiments on tadpoles at Florida State University have demonstrated that there is an embryological connection between olfaction and the brain. For instance, if the left nasal cavity fails to develop properly, so does the left brain hemisphere. A study which was expecting to find increased brain degeneration in rats constantly exposed to odours found the opposite. The control group, breathing non-odorous air, showed *more* degenerative changes. The conclusion was that areas of the brain which get no information may degenerate from disuse. Remember the astronauts on the first long-term space flights? We need odour stimulation for our aesthetic and spiritual well-being. Those few unfortunate enough to have lost their sense of smell altogether find that their life lacks a certain excitement, as if a whole dimension was missing. For them eating becomes merely a task of necessity, almost devoid of pleasure. Most of us have experienced something similar when suffering from a heavy cold.

Although much of the time we are not conscious of odours, the human nose is very sensitive and is capable of distinguishing between hundreds of thousands of different odours and of perceiving quite small amounts of odour. The brain is potentially highly sensitive to smell, although it will not always react fully to odour stimulation. The circumstances of odour research experiments and aromatherapy treatments are very similar and both are designed to induce relaxation and a state of receptivity to odours.

This happy coincidence means that the results of odour research are directly applicable to aromatherapy, while they may not be so applicable to everyday situations in which the brain is being bombarded with other stimuli. In the 'therapeutic situation' of an aromatherapy treatment patients are more receptive to odours, and to the treatment as a whole, than they would be in most other circumstances. As well as being very odour-sensitive, the brain is 'vulnerable' to smells in another sense. They enjoy an immediate access to the brain which is denied to most other remedies or drugs, and there are two distinct reasons for this.

First, smell is the only sense in which the receptor nerve-endings are in *direct* contact with the outside world. To put it another way, your brain extends directly into your nose. There is no equivalent to eyeball or eardrum in between, only a very thin layer of mucus. Smell and touch are our most primitive senses, and so are the most likely to be loaded with instinctive associations, perhaps originating millions of years ago. Of course our other senses have their uses too, but the importance of smell is often not re-cognized. Olfactory nerve cells are the only type of nerve cell in the body which can be replaced if damaged. Pasquale Graziadei, one of the scientists who discovered this pheno-menon, says: 'If you damage a nerve cell of your brain you will never repair it. Blow the neurons in your retina or ear, and you cannot repair the damage. Since olfactory nerve cells can be replaced, the sense of smell has to be very important. Nature never does anything for fun.'[2]

Second, we must consider the blood–brain barrier. The walls of the tiny capillaries that carry blood around the brain are very selective. Although tiny nutrient and oxygen molecules can pass through the capillary walls, larger molecules, including most therapeutic drugs, and blood cannot. Aromatherapy by-passes this 'barrier' by going straight to the brain through the olfactory system. The essential oil itself goes no further than the inside of the nose, but it triggers off a nerve impulse, amplified along the way, which has far-reaching repercussions. Some of the exceptions to the blood–brain barrier rule eloquently reveal the potential power of the 'olfactory by-pass'; for example, the sniffing of glue or cocaine. Cocaine has stimulating effects on the nervous system similar to those of adrenaline. It can cause hallucinations, and habitual use can lead to serious negative personality changes. Even more dramatic is the effect of cyanide. Cyanide kills by preventing the body from utilizing the oxygen in the blood. Taken by mouth it is fatal within two to three minutes. When inhaled it kills within ten seconds.

It is known that a few prescription drugs, including common tranquillizers such as diazepam, *do* get through the blood–brain barrier, and the area of the brain which diazepam affects is the part which controls most of our emotions – the *limbic system*. (As we shall see further on, the limbic system also has special connections with olfaction.) Drugs like diazepam work by interacting with *receptor chemicals* in the brain; without the appropriate receptor they could not work. Susan Schiffman, Professor of Medical Psychology at Duke University, makes an interesting comparison between the action of diazepam and of aromatherapy: 'A group of recently isolated olfactory receptors are the same receptors that bind Valium and Librium [diazepam]. Now, they did not evolve over millions of years so they could be around to bind Valium when it was invented, so why *are* they there in our noses? My guess is that they might be there to bind things that we smell, natural substances that have a similar effect.' [3,4]

It is estimated that three million people in the UK are *addicted* to the group of drugs known as 'minor tranquillizers',

lizers', such as diazepam. Many more take them, but are not addicted. After several years of use the withdrawal symptoms can be as bad as those for heroin addiction. Apart from fatalities, minor tranquillizers cause far more human suffering than does heroin. Is it possible that aromatherapy could offer a natural, and harmless, alternative? Could it even help those who have become addicted to tranquillizers?

I received the following account from Arne Meander, a Danish psychotherapist who has been studying the damaging effects of dependency on tranquillizers. Using a combination of aromatherapy and megavitamin therapy he treated sixteen people in 1986 who had been taking tranquillizers for between six months and twelve years. Meander has concentrated on the main group of minor tranquillizers, the *benzodiazepines*, which include diazepam:

It is obvious that these tranquillizers affect the brain and its activities heavily. After several years of dependency some of the sixteen patients were unable to perform everyday tasks, or to respond to normal communication. The effect is one of depersonalization, a lowering of spiritual awareness, one could almost call it robotism. None of the patients had benefited from the various tranquillizers being taken, but had to continue with them to avoid suffering the effects of withdrawal. After more than twelve months on these drugs, patients experienced some or all of the following side-effects: a lowering of libido; a lowering of appetite and awareness of food quality; a lessening of social contact; a lowering of the ability to fantasize and of mental creativity; a lowering of intellectual capacity, to a degree that they could no longer read a newspaper or tell stories to their children. They were unable to handle any responsibility, and their quality of life as a whole was reduced alarmingly.

To help in the process of withdrawal we used a combination of essential oils such as lavender, melissa, marjoram, ylang-ylang and others, depending on the nature of the individual problem. In some cases it was necessary to make up sedative mixtures to help them sleep at night. The oils were given either orally or by massage. We also used megavitamin therapy, with heavy doses of calcium and magnesium, plus vitamins D, B6, B-complex and minerals. Patients were also given a herbal tea to drink, based on camomile, horsetail, sage, eucalyptus and rosehip. After three weeks on this programme most withdrawal problems cease, and the patient can be 'cleaned out' with the aid of sauna baths and gentle exercise. This has to be done under close supervision, and with the assistance of further aromatherapy and nutrition. I would say it is possible with a holistic approach such as this to rehabilitate anyone who has not suffered severe physical damage from drugs, electric-shock treatment or brain surgery. This general programme was also found to be helpful in the treatment of alcoholism.

Meander makes the comment that treating these patients was very demanding and that initially none of them benefited from massage because they could not feel it. He also found that the essential oils helped the patients to regain their 'spiritual awareness' and so helped them get back in touch with their own inherent healing powers. His three-week programme is impressively short. I have treated one person for alcoholism, and after six months she was greatly improved, but not yet back to normal.

Odour Associations

The human nose protrudes, almost like an antenna, testing the air as we move about and filtering the incoming air. We employ our sense of smell, first to check out, and then to enjoy the food we eat. We even derive pleasure simply from the odour of cooking food, just as we do from perfumes or fragrant flowers. In plants essential oils have two basic functions – attraction and repulsion. The oils frequently act as attractants for certain insects, which then help in the process of fertilization. The oils also protect plants from bacterial infection or from would-be predators. We can see a very similar pattern in man with regard to odours – repulsion linked to danger and attraction linked to procreation. However, in man there is also a new dimension, that of attraction linked purely to pleasure. It is interesting to examine more closely these three primitive reactions to odour.

Warning of danger

In man the repulsion reaction is usually an indication of danger. Rotting food, disease, decay and dampness are invariably injurious to our health and their associated odours are perceived as unpleasant, or 'bad'. The foul odours of fish and rats have given us the sayings: 'There's something fishy going on here' and 'I smell a rat', both of which mean that there is something bad, unpleasant or dangerous which needs uncovering. Other odours perceived by primitive man, such as the smell of an enemy, dangerous animal or burning wood, need to be consciously interpreted. We do not have an instinctive negative reaction to the smell of burning wood because, although fire can indicate danger, it more often indicated 'dinner' or 'warmth' to our ancestors. Consequently such odours are not automatically perceived as unpleasant.

In the insect world chemical odours have very definite meanings and are used as aids to communication. *Iso-amyl acetate* is an aromatic chemical with a powerful, fruity odour and is used in pear flavourings and some perfumes. It occurs naturally in apples and bananas. The same chemical is secreted by a certain type of bee when attacked

by a hornet. This causes other bees to fly out of the hive
and help fight the hornet. To us the smell indicates 'apples'
or 'pears', but to bees it indicates 'Danger, come out and
fight.' According to Francis Bacon the Plague carried with
it a sweet smell, like that of a 'mellow apple'. Certain other
diseases are said to be accompanied by characteristic
odours. In traditional Chinese acupuncture one form of
diagnosis consists of smelling the patient's *subtle* body
odour (not physical body odour). Unpleasant odours have
been used as a form of aversion therapy. Certain sulphurous
odours have been found to dampen the desire for smoking tobacco, and ammonia has been used to suppress
self-injurious behaviour in two hospitalized children.[5]
This type of negative odour conditioning is not a part of
aromatherapy; in fact none of the essential oils are that
unpleasant. However, the success of such conditioning
does demonstrate one way in which odours can influence
behavioural responses.

Sexual signals

In the animal kingdom the female often gives off an
aphrodisiac odour when she is ready for mating. Because
of the way in which human society has evolved, with
monogamy predominating, such advertising is not necessary, although sexual body odours still play an active
role. This is enhanced, sometimes even suppressed, by
the use of perfume. This may seem quite natural and
normal, but why is it that we so often conceal our natural
aphrodisiac body odours and replace them with artificial
aphrodisiac body odours? We do give off aphrodisiac
scents, not only from the genital area, but also in perspiration. The smell of hair, skin and even the breath can
all act as aphrodisiacs, and the effect of such odours is
heightened during sexual intercourse. In aromatherapy

aphrodisiac oils areused to treat impotence, frigidity and similar sexual problems. Many of these oils are also euphoric, counteracting depression and evoking a feeling of well-being. There are also a few antiaphrodisiac oils, known as *anaphrodisiacs*, like oil of marjoram. Both these and the aphrodisiac oils all have other uses in aromatherapy, and by no means do they always have an influence on sexual feelings.

Enjoyment

Civilized man has lost some of the more practical uses of the sense of smell, such as sniffing out an enemy or tracking an animal, but has greatly developed the aesthetic, pleasurable aspect. Odour and enjoyment are most commonly linked in foods and fragrances. Connoisseurs of wine understand the importance of smell, or 'bouquet', in the appreciation of a vintage wine. In fact what we think of as our sense of taste is about 80 per cent smell. We can only taste sweet, salty, sour and bitter, and we rely on the subtle sensitivities of our noses to impart those nuances of 'flavour' which modern man has invested so much energy in developing. We have also combined the concept of aphrodisiac odours with the pleasure derived from smelling a fragrant flower to create what we call a 'perfume', which embodies enjoyment and attraction at the same time. This 'pleasure connection' has now been taken to a further level of sophistication (largely for commercial reasons) with the use of fine fragrances in room fresheners, shampoos, soaps and many other everyday consumer items. Odours are even being used subliminally, because it has been found that consumers will prefer a scented product to an identical unscented one, even though the fragrance is not consciously perceived.

Odour Conditioning

Are odours subconsciously associated with behavioural responses? A study to answer this question was carried out at Warwick University in 1983.[6] The experiment was split into two parts, and at no time did the subjects understand the nature of the study. In the first part they were deliberately put into a stressful situation; they were asked to complete a timed task requiring manual dexterity as well as logical thought. Unknown to the subjects an odour, trimethylundecyclenic aldehyde (TUA), was impregnated on the instruction sheet pinned to the board in front of them. The dilution was such that subjects were not consciously aware of the odour. Afterwards they were asked if they would like to participate in a different experiment being run by someone else at the University.

The second part took place three days later and showed conclusively that a significant degree of stress could be induced in the same subjects by exposing them to low concentrations of the same odour. They had been conditioned to associate this particular odour with a stress situation. When they were later given TUA to smell, and asked if they had smelt it before, very few thought they had.

I once read that aromatherapy could not possibly amount to very much because the human nose habituates quite quickly to odours. After a few minutes we cannot smell essential oils any more and so therefore they are no longer having any effect. This is absolutely untrue, as the Warwick study demonstrates. Odours do affect us, even if we do not consciously perceive them. Sometimes people find the concept of 'therapeutic aromas' difficult to accept, but this is not surprising if our conscious mind is frequently unaware of the presence of odours. Even when we do notice smells, we often do not realize that we are being affected in some way.

In another study subjects were given two types of paint to test, not knowing that the only difference was in the odour. The perfumed paint was said by the subjects to cover better and to go on more smoothly than the unperfumed one. One of the major fragrance companies conducted a study in which subjects were asked to compare two rooms. They were identical in every detail, except that one of the rooms contained a low level of fragrance. The fragrant room was described as being brighter, cleaner and fresher, but not one person noticed the presence of the fragrance.[3]

In all three of these studies the odours were present at levels perceptible to the human nose, but our *conscious* brain frequently does not register the presence of an odour until it becomes quite strong. When the presence of the odour was pointed out to subjects after an experiment, they were then able to smell it. We may feel that such tests are unfair in a sense, and make people seem stupid, but in fact the subjects *did notice a difference*, but they interpreted it in non-olfactory terms. In the Warwick test there was a response to odour presence, but it was on a subconscious level.

Olfaction and Memory

There are several ways in which olfaction and memory are related. Claims that certain essential oils have the capacity to stimulate memory and concentration can be traced back to the first century A D. Among the most potent essences in this connection are basil, peppermint and rosemary (see pp. 183–5), all essential oils with strong, piercing odours. I do not refer to the stimulation of particular memories, perhaps by association with one of these odours, but to improving the capacity to remember – to remember anything at all. This is closely related to learning, much of which is based on our ability to memorize facts. Concentration is also tied up with memory and learning. If you find concentration difficult then your ability to learn, in the sense of memorizing, is going to be impaired.

If we accept that some essential oils are stimulants of the central nervous system (see p. 138) then it makes complete sense to postulate that they can increase our capacity to focus and to concentrate our minds. This, in turn, could easily lead to an improvement in our capacity to remember things. Until very recently any claims that essential oils could improve memory were treated as nothing more than old wives' tales. However, odour researchers in universities around the world are now making very similar claims themselves. We now know that an area of the brain known as the *limbic system* contains the main centres both for memory and olfaction. These centres, then, are not found close to each other, they are *the same areas*.

Howard Ehrlichman, of City University, New York, constructed a test to examine the connection between memory, emotion and odour. He isolated subjects in a bare, almost dark room, the only item in the room being a picture hanging on a wall. An odour was then released into the air and the subjects were asked to relate which memories were stirred up. He deliberately used odours which would be either pleasant or unpleasant. Those who smelled the pleasant odours recalled pleasant, positive memories, such as making new friends or a day out on the town. Those who experienced the unpleasant smells tended to recall unhappy situations, such as periods of pain. These are *general* odour memories, rather than *specific* ones. The memories were not stimulated *directly* by the odours, but subconscious associations were made between pleasant odour and pleasant memory, or unpleasant odour and unpleasant memory.

Specific odour memories are much more personal, and will vary from one person to another, but such memories are often remarkably strong. It has been demonstrated that long-term odour memory is stronger than long-term visual memory, as illustrated in Figure 8.[7] This would seem to indicate that there is an important reason why we should preserve our smell–memory associations. It may be to do with self-preservation. An animal which eats something which makes it ill is not likely to ever eat the same thing again.

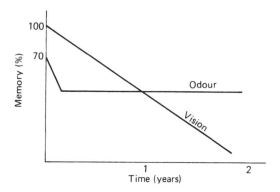

Figure 8. Olfactory and visual memory over time.

Unpleasant odour associations are often unwanted, but not easy to get rid of. There was the lady who purchased a new and expensive perfume in a New York department store. Later the same day, wearing her new perfume, she was in an elevator when most of the city was hit by an electrical power failure. Having spent some twelve hours in the elevator, along with her new perfume, she could not bear to wear it again, since it made her feel claustrophobic. Most of us would not consider the smell of diesel oil to be a pleasant one, but for one woman it always brings back memories of her very happy, early years of marriage. Her husband had worked on the railways, and she would welcome him home in the evening, with him smelling strongly of diesel oil. Individual odour associations are learned ones, acquired during our lifetimes, and have little bearing on aromatherapy. Pleasant associations with essential oils being used in therapy will only help to enhance the positive effects of treatment. However, any unpleasant associations (I have never come across any) would be best avoided by using a different essential oil.

If essential oils can stimulate memory, or even memories, it would seem a logical treatment for any type of memory defect such as amnesia, although I do not know of any examples of this. Coma is another problem condition which may respond to aromatherapy. According to a 1986 report in the French *Vogue* magazine,[8] a group of doctors on the West Coast of the USA are using odours to treat comatose patients. The article also quotes a story by Jeff Miles, executive of a fragrance company, whose grandfather was a perfumer. Apparently his grandfather fell into a coma and did not recover for five weeks. A nurse would bathe him every day, and his first reaction while recovering consciousness one day during his bath was to the smell of the jasmine soap she used. (One cannot help wondering, however, whether touch may also have played some part in the man's recovery.)

Another case of coma recovery was attributed to peppermint oil. In October 1983 a seventeen-year-old boy from Herefordshire, England, was involved in an accident while riding his bicycle. After lying comatose in a hospital bed for three months he regained consciousness after smelling peppermint oil. He still suffers from slight brain damage, but owes his recovery to his father, who tried the peppermint oil because his son had always been fond of mints. Whether recovery was due purely to memory association, or whether the peppermint also had some brain-stimulating effect, we cannot say, but the possibilities for aromatherapy in such otherwise hopeless cases seem worth pursuing.

Olfaction and the Brain

Although we still do not know exactly how the nose perceives odour, we do know where it takes place. At the top of the inner nasal cavity, level with the bridge of the nose, are two areas of special mucous membrane about the size of a thumb-nail. This special lining tissue is covered in a very thin layer of mucus, and is known as *olfactory epithelium*. Into the mucus layer protrude some 20 million of tiny hairs which are in fact the endings of small olfactory nerves. These tiny hairs somehow translate odour into a nerve message which then travels along the small nerve and into one of the two main olfactory nerves. The aromatic vapour itself travels no further than the nose, and is breathed out again (some is absorbed by the lungs). However, the odour triggers off a nerve message which is capable of intricate and far-reaching repercussions.

From the two main olfactory nerves the message passes into a section of the brain known as the *limbic system* (L S) (see Figure 9). This is sometimes referred to as the 'old brain' and was one of the first parts to develop in our ancestors, some seventy million years ago. (The cortex, the outer part of the brain which performs intellectual functions, developed later on.) The anatomy books show the intimate connection between the L S and the olfactory nerves,[9] and the old name for the L S was *rhinencephalon*, meaning smell-brain. We know the L S is a complex series of structures, and we know that one of them, the piriform area, has to do with the conscious perception of odour, but what about the rest of it? According to Dr Van Toller of the Olfaction Research Group at Warwick University it comprises thirty-four structures and fifty-three pathways.[10] Why should the incoming messages from the nose be linked up to such a complex system, when only one of the structures is known to perform the obvious function of registering smell? Could it be because our brains are wired to respond to odours in complex, subtle ways which are, as yet, little understood? But we do know a little about the

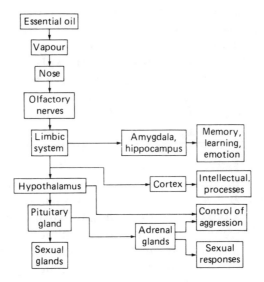

Figure 9. The relationship between olfaction, memory, emotion and mood.

L S; we know, for instance, that it is strongly linked to *emotional* responses.

Stimulation of the L S of animals results in either pleasure or pain, depending on the exact area stimulated. Other studies have shown that animals respond by either becoming very aggressive or very docile – again, opposing responses.[9] Valnet reports a study in which oils of fennel or rosemary made animals apprehensive, while wormwood, hyssop or sage caused them to become aggressive.[11] There are anecdotal reports that oils of clary sage and ylang-ylang make dogs docile (see p. 198). According to anatomists the L S plays a major role in many emotions, including pleasure, pain, rage, docility, anger, fear, sorrow, affection and sexual feelings.[9]

The two parts of the L S which are frequently referred to in the literature are the *hippocampus* and the *amygdala*. They are said to be very much involved in both emotion and memory, and they are certainly involved with olfaction, since they both receive nerve fibres from the olfactory nerves. Here we can see an anatomical explanation of how odours could stimulate memory or memories, and certain emotions. Exactly what is evoked will depend on the odour, so different essential oils could evoke either intellectual arousal (concentration), emotional arousal (euphoria, affection) or sexual arousal. The essential oils do not appear to evoke negative responses.

I believe that highly synthetic odours, ones which do not occur in nature, are being researched for para-military use. These are odours which evoke feelings such as revulsion, fear and a strong desire to flee, to escape the odour. I once had the opportunity to smell one of these odours in great dilution. While I did not run out of the building, as others have apparently done, I experienced a most unpleasant feeling, one I would not wish on anyone. I suppose winning a battle by means of odour is preferable to using bullets and bombs. Fragrance fights actually do happen in the animal kingdom. Opposing groups of lemur monkeys have what is known as a 'ritual stink fight'. They wipe their tails under their armpits, turn their backs to each other and waft their tails in the air. The smelliest group wins and the other retreats.

Another unique feature of the sense of smell is that the olfactory nerves do not cross over to the opposite side of the brain. Our brains are almost completely divided into two 'hemispheres' – left and right. It is generally accepted now that the left hemisphere is more concerned with logical thought processes and verbalization, and the right with intuitive, creative thought. It is a curious fact that smell messages from the left nostril travel, via the left olfactory nerve, to the left, logical side of the brain. Smells picked up by the right nostril mainly affect the right, intuitive side.

In 1969 and 1974 some interesting studies were conducted with people who had previously undergone surgery to separate the left and right hemispheres (though not for the purpose of this study!).[12] This operation makes the distinction between left nostril/hemisphere and right nostril/hemisphere even more clear. In these studies the subjects had no trouble in naming odours presented to their left nostrils, but had great difficulty naming odours presented to their right nostrils. The right side of the brain would react to odour more emotionally – like/dislike, aesthetic appreciation – but would have found a logical interpretation, such as naming the odour, much more difficult. For the left hemisphere odour identification would present no problem, assuming the smell was a familiar one.

It has also been suggested that the right hemisphere is more involved than the left in the feeling known as 'euphoria', and also in the functions of imagination and pleasure. This would explain the importance of olfaction in inducing altered states of consciousness in religious and creative rituals. This important relationship between olfaction and the right hemisphere also helps to explain the ability of aromatherapy to induce euphoria and a consequent distancing from anxieties. Essential oils would appear to be ideal psychotherapeutic 'drugs'. Unlike the minor tranquillizers they promote creative thought and pleasant feelings, instead of suppressing them, and of course are completely non-addictive.

It is known that certain parts of the cortex are related to sight, hearing, speech and so on. So far no cortical area has been found corresponding to smell, and we do not know whether such an area exists or not. However, some very recent experiments by Van Toller show that when we smell something the *whole* of the cortex may be stimulated.[10] With the aid of computer technology he has been able to show a video image of the subject's cortex at the same time as they inhale an odour. In less than one second the computerized image shows areas of colour lighting up in different parts of the cortex, each colour indicating a degree of stimulation. In the illustration (Figure 10) the right hemisphere is showing a higher level of activity than the left, showing that the subject is experiencing relaxed pleasure from a pleasant odour. Any confusion or intense thought would have shown up as increased activity on the left side, which is very placid in this particular case.

We know that people respond to odours quite strongly: we either like them or we do not – the like/dislike response. In 1983 Van Toller[13] showed that dislike of an odour leads to rejection – we block it out. His study demonstrates that odours perceived as unpleasant produce less response from the nervous system, and he makes the point that pleasant and unpleasant responses should not be regarded as oppo-

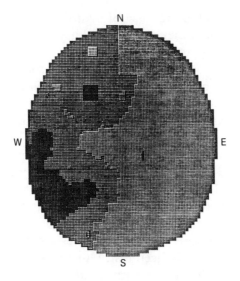

Figure 10. A computerized brain scan, showing the outer layers of the brain from above, taken five seconds after the subject was given a pleasant odour to smell. The right hemisphere (lighter shade) shows about twice as much activity as the left. (Reproduced by kind permission of Dr Van Toller, Warwick Olfaction Research Group)

sites. Pleasant odours gain a deeper access to our nervous systems, because we do not block them. This lends support to the notion that pleasant therapies are sometimes more beneficial than unpleasant ones, an approach first put into practice by Asclepiades over 2000 years ago. It also ties in with the discovery by Rovesti that psychiatric patients show very much more improvement under the influence of pleasant odours than unpleasant ones.[14] From my own experience of aromatherapy I find that the more fragrant essential oils, such as rose and ylang-ylang, are more capable of producing a positive emotional response than, say, eucalyptus or tea-tree. However, I would hesitate to condone the use of synthetic perfumes in this context, although their commercial use as evokers of mood is, I am sure, quite harmless.

It seems probable that we have what could be called a 'layered response' to odours. First, we either accept or reject – the like/dislike response. Then the two hemispheres respond separately – the left intellectually (odour description/identification) and the right creatively. The right brain response may then give rise to a deeper emotional/hormonal reaction, and perhaps beyond the left brain response may lie a personal memory association. This is all conjecture, and even if there is such a pattern it may vary from situation to situation. As the human brain has evolved over millions of years the primitive odour responses associated with the L S have not entirely been lost. Our aesthetic appreciation of odours is also tied in with instinctive reactions which rarely reach our conscious mind and with emotional reactions which we sometimes cannot identify or explain. In the words of Van Toller: 'At each level of brain development the functions of emotion and olfaction have been carried forward and incorporated into the newly evolved neural structures, each progressive step adding new dimensions and broadening the original functions in subtle ways.'

It has been claimed recently that all our emotions are the result of certain chemicals being released into the bloodstream. One cannot help feeling (or is it thinking?) that there is more to feeling romantic than a little *phenylethylamine* tugging at one's nerve endings. The interplay between thought and feeling is complex, and there is no space to go into it here, but emotion, thought, mood and olfaction are all closely related. The neurochemical–emotional connection has now been quite well established, so it is worth mentioning that essential oils also stimulate the release of neurochemicals, as well as hormones, in the body. Massage is capable of similar effects, so it is not surprising that aromatherapy makes you feel good. The fact that essential oils cause the body to release its own 'drugs' goes a long way to explaining why they are capable of harmless, subtle, yet powerful effects.

Aromatherapy and Emotion

The following account, which dates from 1985, is from an occupational therapist who was then working at the Merrifield Children's Unit in Taunton, Devon.

I use essential oils in conjunction with foot reflexology [see p. 153] to promote relaxation in emotionally disturbed children. I try to involve the children in their own treatment, and hope that they will recognize and to some extent become responsible for their feelings. I usually 'go by the nose', especially after a little epileptic girl picked out the only anticonvulsive oil I had as her favourite. I also discovered that lavender and ylang-ylang worked a miracle for a school-phobic child who had to take a French oral exam. She later recommended it to a medical student, whose sister got exam nerves. I must confess I have tried it myself and it certainly helped.

I have found that some of the oils, especially rosemary, help to bring back memories – some pleasant, some painful – but at least they can be talked about. Marjoram oil has a definite effect on grief. A very homesick child reacted well, as did another, who was grieving for a lost pet. Geranium is the one chosen most often by patients with *anorexia nervosa*, and lavender is very effective for insomnia; the children ask for pillow pets filled with it. Clary sage oil seems to have a beneficial effect in hyperactive children, and I have noted its effect as an antidepressant and sedative.

In December 1923 two Italian doctors, Giovanni Gatti and Renato Cayola, published an article entitled: 'The action of essences on the nervous system'.[15] It was the first study of its kind to be published. The authors gave subjects pads of cotton wool to sniff, these having been impregnated with one of several essential oils. Another method used was to spray the surrounding air with solutions of the oils. The two doctors discuss the opposing states of anxiety and depression, and the use of sedative oils for the former and of stimulating oils for the latter. In this particular study they were not treating patients suffering from such problems, but were simply looking for either a stimulating or sedative response. Changes were noted and measured in pulse rate, blood circulation and depth of respiration immediately following essential oil inhalation.

Essential oils identified as sedatives, and therefore of use in anxiety states, include orange blossom, orange leaf (petitgrain), melissa, chamomile, cedarwood and valerian. Ylang-ylang is the only one recommended for depression. It is also described as an aphrodisiac, although no reason is given for saying this. They conclude that the sense of smell has, by reflex action, an enormous influence on the function of the central nervous system.

This early research has been taken a stage further in recent years by Rovesti, another Italian.[14,16] He also recommends inhalation as the means of application, usually by spraying the air with aromatic aerosols. He gives no details of the studies carried out, but states that: 'Very conclusive experiments have been carried out in various clinics for nervous diseases, on patients affected by hysteria or psychic depression.' He comments that mixtures of essential oils are more pleasant, and therefore more acceptable than single oils for those suffering from nervous tension. For depression he lists jasmine, sandalwood, orange, ylang-ylang, verbena and lemon; and for anxiety bergamot, orange blossom, cypress, lavender, orange leaf, lime, rose, violet leaf and marjoram. Rovesti has taken matters one stage further than Gatti and Cayola, by actually using aromatherapy on people suffering from psychological disturbances. He comments: 'It may be said that the patients feel as if transported by the essential oil into a different, more agreeable and acceptable world, so that many of their reactive instincts are curbed and they gradually return towards normality.'

Smelling a fragrant flower makes you feel good inside, and aromatherapy has the same effect. From the initial like/dislike response to an odour there may be a variety of emotional effects. We have already seen that the nerve stimulants are useful in depressive states, and the nerve sedatives for anxiety. We have also seen that the evocative power of odours, known since ancient times, has been utilized in religious ceremony, alchemical practices and magic, as well as in healing. It has also been employed in seduction. Aromatics have been very widely used in love potions and aphrodisiacs for centuries. Apart from their obvious personal use, the sexually stimulating properties of essential oils can help those who suffer from impotence or frigidity. Both of these are known to be largely emotional in origin, which therefore demonstrates that the oils have some effect on the emotions. The aphrodisiac effect of ylang-ylang oil has already been alluded to.

Feeling good, and feeling sexually aroused, are linked, though different. We have already seen that the L S and the right cerebral hemisphere, both areas of the brain related to smell response, have been linked with the feeling known as *euphoria*. This simply means feeling good, high, on top of the world, and euphoric essential oils, such as clary sage, are employed in the treatment of depression. Some depressions are passing moods, and some are much more serious. I do not want to give the impression that a quick whiff of clary sage oil is all that is needed. However, I have had a great deal of success in treating depressive people by applying my own principles of holistic aromatherapy (see p. 142). It is interesting that some of the most effective euphoric oils happen to be aphrodisiacs too – jasmine, ylang-ylang and clary sage especially.

Application

Many studies have demonstrated that essential oils are capable of sedative effects when given internally. However, the dosage required to obtain significant sedation is very high – about 100 times greater than the amounts actually used in aromatherapy.[17] Such elevated dosage is potentially hazardous. Sedation, and other psychotherapeutic effects, can be achieved with much smaller amounts when the oils are inhaled. This simple fact has been known empirically for thousands of years but was not investigated until recently. In 1921 Macht set out to investigate the possibility that aromatics could 'exert their therapeutic effects, not by being first absorbed into the circulation, but through a direct stimulation of the olfactory sense organs'. Results showed that certain aromatics, when inhaled, have distinct sedative effects on rats.[18]

Evidence of a similar effect on human subjects comes from a recent Japanese study.[19] Professor Shizuo Torii, from Toho University, set out to distinguish between stimulating and sedative essential oils. As his measuring device he used a particular brainwave known as contingent negative variation (CNV), which is a wave created by anticipation. To begin with, two essences were investigated – jasmine, thought to be a stimulant, and lavender, known for its sedative action. Electrodes attached to the head of subjects picked up and recorded the brainwaves. Subjects were given a simple task to perform, which created a state of anticipation, and they were then given an essential oil to smell. The CNV wave, or 'anticipation wave', either increased or decreased depending on the essential oil being smelled. This indicated, respectively, either nervous stimulation or sedation. The results are shown in Figure 11, in which the significant part of the curves are where they cross the dotted area. The first one shows a normal reading; the second, after inhalation of jasmine, shows stimulation; the third, after inhalation of lavender shows sedation.

Torii carried out further studies on a number of essential oils which, in 80 per cent of cases, agreed with the result

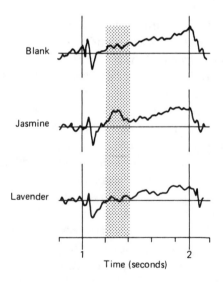

Blank

Jasmine

Lavender

1   2
Time (seconds)

Figure 11. Three CNV wave readings. The response occurs less than one second after inhalation. (After a photograph by Professor Shizuo Torii, Toho University School of Medicine)

expected from empirical knowledge. In practice it is found that olfaction on its own is less effective than it is when combined with counselling, creative visualization or massage.

Primal memory

The fragrance that came to each was like a memory of dewy mornings, of unshadowed sun, of which the fair world in spring is but a fleeting memory.

J. R. R. Tolkien, *The Lord of the Rings*

Since the influence of odour on both memory and emotion is so closely related could it be that odours evoke the memory of emotions? Could aromatherapy evoke half-buried feelings from childhood, perhaps pure feelings of joy, wonder, selfless, innocent love and warmth? Perhaps such deep feelings are even somehow related to primitive, instinctive feelings which have been ingrained in the human soul for hundreds of thousands of years. If this were true then smelling an essential oil for the first time might well elicit a strong feeling like that of *déjà vu*. I have witnessed exactly this when giving essential oils to seminar delegates, patients or aromatherapy students. 'It reminds me of something but I cannot put my finger on it' is the typical, frustrated response. Other explanations are possible for this, but I leave the reader to make up their own mind.

It is evident that natural odours are necessary for our optimum spiritual well-being. It is also clear that pleasant odours in themselves are not as effective as essential oils used in a therapeutic context. You can bottle essential oils, but not aromatherapy.

Some case studies

Anxiety and asthma (therapist: Sandra Staplehurst)

Peter first came to see me in February 1986 when he was forty-seven years old. He had suffered from asthma since early childhood, and had a long list of allergies, but the main problem he wanted help with was what he described as his 'edginess' with people close to him and his eruptions of temper. This edgy feeling was accompanied by an inflamed red patch on his chest at times of most stress and by a twitch in his left shoulder and eye. He had received psychiatric treatment for his asthma in 1970, but had never had any previous bodywork therapy. Considering his character type I decided to use camomile. Being a very 'watery' oil it would counteract what I felt to be a slightly unhealthy interest in the sensual pleasures, and would help to put him more in touch with his emotions. The camomile was most often combined with sandalwood and ylang-ylang, both of which would help to slow him down and relieve his anxiety. I massaged his chest and back on alternate weeks.

The difference in Peter after the first treatment was immediate. He reported that the edginess and temper disappeared like magic. He was undergoing a great deal of stress in his relationship with his girlfriend at the time. Although she was not well, and was very depressive, he found that he did not react by being edgy with her any longer, and consequently she was also improving. They used the oils in fragrances, and he used the mixtures from his massages in between visits. After a few months of treatment Peter said that they had decided to get married. As he had changed so much she now felt happy about living with him permanently, and he with her, despite the fact that he had lived alone for seventeen years. Four months after his first treatment Peter was married, although he continued to come for weekly treatments.

His choice of essential oils is now much lighter. Melissa has become a favourite, and we no longer use any of the three original oils. He regards the treatment as ongoing therapy, and feels that he needs it to cope with the stress of his work. His emotional life is much more stable and he very rarely has an attack of asthma now. He feels that the aromatherapy has helped him to identify his own problems of reacting to stress, and to remain calm. His allergic reactions have greatly diminished, and he can now tolerate some of the things he had to avoid previously. It is now nine months since his first visit. His wife's health has also improved, and Peter says that I am treating 'two for the price of one', although I never see her.

Anxiety/depression (therapist: Robert Tisserand)

Mrs W. came to see me complaining of depression, which she said had started following a hysterectomy operation fourteen years before. She also suffered from headaches and dizzy spells almost every day and was not sleeping well. She had been taking tranquillizers for four years, but had stopped taking them six years ago. A likeable but very timid person in her early forties, she was married and had three children. She was very much lacking in confidence, and said that her mother had told her, ever since she was very young, that she had been an unwanted baby. Even now her mother still mentioned this periodically.

Oriental diagnosis showed that she had many weaknesses in her subtle energy system, especially over the lower abdominal area. I mixed up a blend of basil, bergamot, clary sage and geranium, which was used in massage once a week, and I encouraged her, in a very simple way, to be more assertive and self-confident. A week after her first treatment she was sleeping better and reported having only three dizzy spells and no headaches at all.

After three weeks she had had only two days of headache and depression and was generally more energetic, brighter and a little more confident. At this point I changed the essential oil blend, but otherwise we continued as before. By the seventh week her depression seemed no more than a distant memory, which in itself gave her an enormous boost. However, she still showed some subtle energy weaknesses and I advised her to stop eating chocolate and yeast as there was a probable allergy to these. After sixteen weeks she no longer felt any need for treatment. Her depression and dizzy spells had gone and she was only having mild headaches once every two to three weeks. Her general energy level, confidence and quality of sleep had greatly improved and she felt much more at ease with herself.

Depression/nightmares (therapist: Robert Tisserand)

Mrs A., seventy-two years old, had lost her husband and one of her three children, who died from a heroin overdose. She was very fit for her age and was a basically cheerful person, but she did suffer from increasing periods of depression. She also revealed that she had been experiencing nightmares every night for the past month or so. She lived alone and would wake up every morning in a cold sweat feeling terrified. The cause of these problems seemed to stem from the death of her son. She ate a very healthy diet and took one sleeping tablet every night to help her sleep.

I gave her whole-body massage, using a blend of frankincense, bergamot, clary sage and jasmine. During the first week following treatment she had a few strange dreams, but no nightmares at all. I think I was even more pleased than she about this, since I did not know of a remedy for nightmares as such, but had simply prescribed oils according to her subtle energy weaknesses. During the following three weeks she made steady progress, with no further nightmares. She reported feeling much better in herself and her cloud of depression gradually dispersed. By the end of this period she had stopped taking the nightly sleeping pill, as she found she could now do without it.

The following week was the anniversary of her son's death and she had three bad nightmares, all involving him. However, she did not go back to the pills and came through this almost inevitable relapse very well. After a further three weeks she was very much improved. She still showed some subtle energy weakness, but had had no more nightmares and felt able to carry on without the support of aromatherapy.

CHAPTER SIX

THE TREATMENT

Massage enables the patient to see his illness in new ways, to obtain insight into his condition, and to want to learn more about his own contribution to recovery.

Georg Groddeck

If you are going to go to an aromatherapist for treatment you will want to find a good one. If you have been impressed by what you have read so far you will want to find someone who has been trained as a holistic therapist. There are two aromatherapy associations (see p. 210) which have lists of recommended therapists. If you cannot find a *recommended* therapist within striking distance, you are entitled to ask a few questions before you make an appointment, and a list of suggestions to help you follows.

* Do they have a bona fide qualification *in aromatherapy*? (This will usually be a diploma rather than a certificate, and it is essential that they have this.)
* Are they a *full* member of an aromatherapy association?
* How long was their aromatherapy training? (If it was less than several months they are unlikely to be competent, even if they had some previous medical knowledge.)
* Do they blend their own oils and make up individual prescriptions for each patient? This is an essential requirement.
* Is aromatherapy a sideline for them, or do they specialize in it?

Personal recommendation is usually a good indication.

Some useful advice when having aromatherapy treatment

Allergy to perfume

A few people are allergic to perfume ingredients and find that virtually any perfume will cause a minor rash where it is applied to the skin. If you are one of these people there is a very good chance that you will not be able to tolerate essential oils either. Another therapy, perhaps homoeopathy or acupuncture, would be more suitable for you, at least while the allergy lasts. Most perfume ingredients, and most essential oils, have the potential to cause very slight skin irritation. They have no effect on most of us, but those with a hypersensitivity will react.

What to expect from treatment

There are no guarantees in any kind of medicine. Although dramatic improvements and 'miracle cures' do happen, and it is wonderful when they do, they are the exception rather than the rule. Do not expect your therapist to be able to predict exactly how many treatments you will require to reach a certain level of improvement. 'Cure' is a word very rarely used in alternative medicine, because we recognize that the background, or underlying cause, of a condition is hardly ever *completely* eradicated, even though symptoms may disappear. The rate of improvement will vary from one individual to another, and in general this will be slower with age. Most therapists reckon that the longer you have had a condition the longer it will take to 'cure'.

Ideally you should expect a steady improvement from week to week, and I think it is fair to say that you should feel better to some degree after your first treatment. Initially the kind of feedback I generally get is 'I am sleeping much better' or 'I have more energy' or 'My appetite has improved' or 'The ache is not so bad' or 'I feel brighter in myself'. These are the first signs of healing, and although they may appear to be unimportant they are very significant. They show that the treatment is already starting to take effect. If you do experience wonderful results after the first one or two treatments that is fine, but do not expect the same after *every* treatment, or you might be disappointed!

'Reactions'

If your symptoms generally worsen from week to week, then something is very wrong. However, sometimes people do experience a temporary worsening of symptoms, often after the first or second treatment. This may take the form of a headache, a lowering of energy levels, increase in aches and pains or a depression. A typical reaction will come on within twenty-four hours of the treatment *and will not last more than a day or two*. It is invariably followed by the opposite reaction – you feel very much better. This may not happen to you at all, but if it does, and you are worried about it, do contact your therapist.

In the long run, whether it is weeks, months or even years, your condition will, I hope, improve. To maintain this state of health it is a good idea to have regular 'maintenance' treatments, perhaps once every three months. Those who lead very hectic lives, or have high pressure work or home situations, do find that weekly or monthly aromatherapy treatment helps to maintain their energy levels, helps them to cope with the physical and mental stresses of modern life.

As you have probably realized by now you can expect an *overall* improvement, not just one in your major complaint.

How you can help

Aromatherapists have put a lot of time and energy into their training, and invest much care and effort in each treatment, which is a unique personal experience for them, as well as for you. You can help yourself considerably by following the guidelines below.

Your attitude

For some this is by far the most important piece of advice in the whole book. If you are sick and you want to get well you must learn to *help yourself*, to heal yourself, to love yourself and you must be *determined* to get well. A negative or couldn't-care-less-about-myself attitude is the most difficult hurdle for both you and your therapist to overcome. In the Aquarian Gospel Jesus says: 'But the greatest healer of all is he who can inspire faith' – faith in *yourself*.

A story reported in the *Journal of Alternative Medicine*, August 1986, tells of two men both ill in hospital in the USA. By accident their medical files were switched. The result was that doctors told a man terminally sick with cancer that he would soon be better, while his neighbour, who only had a minor recoverable illness, was told he had just two months to live. The man with cancer was soon up and about and apparently completely well, while the mildly ill man promptly died, almost exactly two months later!

Whether true or not, it is a very believable story, and certainly would seem to shed some doubt on the wisdom of 'giving it straight' to terminal or very sick patients. Believing that you can get better can do nothing but help and it is not a *substitute* for therapy. If you can heal yourself by faith alone, fantastic, but the chances are that you will need all the help you can get.

Follow advice

This is all tied up with helping yourself. Your therapist may not ask you to do anything, but you may be asked to change your diet in some way, to do certain exercises, to take certain remedies, or nutritional supplements, to cut down on alcohol, coffee, or cigarettes. If you honestly feel that your therapist is asking too much of you, then say so, and try to reach a compromise. However, if at all possible try to follow the advice, after all, it is for your own good.

Perfume

Unless your therapist advises otherwise it is fine for you to wear perfume, cologne, aftershave or any other fragrance *except* on the day of your treatment. Apart from clashing with the essential oil blend used by your therapist a strong perfume could feasibly interfere with the effect of the oils on the nervous system. If you are using massage oils or bath oils at home, made up by your aromatherapist, abstention from fragrances is advisable. However, if this is causing you social problems, do discuss it with your therapist.

Bathing

Taking a bath or shower before going for treatment is fine, although try not to use a highly scented soap. Your therapist will certainly love you the more if you do wash before your visit and it will also help you to get into a relaxed state. However, after your massage do *not* take a bath or shower for at least six hours because you will wash off the very oils that your body needs. After treatment a very fine layer of oil remains on the skin and is slowly absorbed into the system. Also, do not use talcum powder or anything else on your skin after your pre-treatment bath. Talc, especially, blocks the pores and will hinder absorption of the essential oils.

Sunbathing

Sunbathing after a treatment is not advisable for two reasons. First it is energy-sapping, and that is just what you do not need at this time. Second there could be a reaction between the oils on your skin and the sun. This is why you should never wear perfume when going under a sun-bed. Sun-beds should also be avoided after a treatment. The next day you may lie in the sun to your heart's content.

Alcohol

You will undo some of the benefit gained from your treatment if you drink heavily on the day of your treatment. A little alcohol is fine, but stay sober.

Rest afterwards

Do not 'squeeze in' an aromatherapy treatment in the middle of a busy day. Work beforehand by all means, but do allow yourself plenty of time to rest afterwards. At this point you are in a sensitive, fragile state. Some physical and/or emotional problems may have been 'stirred up' and the best thing you can do is to relax and take things easy. You may feel disorientated for a short time and will probably feel tired for a couple of hours afterwards. Also you may have a 'reaction', so do not do anything that is going to make great demands on your energy. You need this time for yourself, eitheto 'recover' from your treatment or simply to enjoy your new-found energy.

The Consultation

The first time you visit an aromatherapist, even if you have nothing very much wrong with you, there will be some kind of consultation. You will be asked the kind of questions all natural therapists ask. First, your personal details – name, address, age, occupation, etc.; and then all about your complaint – when it started, when and how it bothers you, details of any previous treatment and so on. Also, the aromatherapist will want to know something about your previous medical history – any accidents, operations or serious illnesses – and about your general health. This means your diet, the amount of exercise you do, your consumption of tobacco and alcohol and any allergies or other minor complaints you might have. You will also be asked about any mental or emotional stresses in your life, although you are not obliged to talk about anything if you do not want to. However, most people are under stress of some sort – to do with relationships, money, work or something similar. Stresses, whether they are emotional, mental, physical, nutritional or environmental, all have an effect on our total state of health and well-being.

Aromatherapists do not have a thorough training in clinical diagnosis and if this is needed they will have to rely on the opinion of a doctor or other medical practitioner (e.g. medical herbalist). Clinical diagnosis means being able to diagnose a condition from the physical symptoms present, and perhaps also from tests, such as urine or blood analysis. It includes the activities we commonly associate with our general practitioner, such as taking blood pressure, listening to the heart and looking into the ears or throat. Even a general practitioner will not always know right away what the problem is and may refer a patient to another doctor or specialist for a second opinion. And, as we all know, doctors are human and sometimes do make an incorrect diagnosis.

There is another type of diagnosis, which I will call *holistic* diagnosis, and which is learned and practised by natural therapists. There are many aspects to it, but basically it identifies what we could call areas of *weakness* in the body, as opposed to specific diseases. While clinical diagnosis might identify the presence of a disease such as 'chronic bronchitis', holistic diagnosis might conclude that the lungs, large intestine and kidneys all show signs of weakness. Another person, also with chronic bronchitis, might show a different pattern, perhaps a weakness in the heart and lungs. Because of the obvious physical symptoms we would always expect the lungs to show some kind of weakness. However, other weak areas, not revealed by clinical diagnosis, would also need attention *as well* as the lungs, and it could be a different pattern of weaknesses every time. This is what we mean when we talk about treating the person as an individual. Incidentally, these 'secondary weaknesses' may or may not be detectable by clinical diagnosis, depending on how much the physical organ is actually affected. A weakness, especially in the early stages, is too subtle to result in any obvious physical problem, and so a 'weak heart', for example, in holistic terms, might not be anything to worry about.

How does holistic diagnosis work? There are quite a number of techniques which come under this heading. Some of the principal ones are described below.

Oriental Diagnosis

Not commonly used by aromatherapists, this is mentioned here because it relates to the next item, 'touch for health'. Oriental diagnosis is not easy to summarize as it is rather complex. It is normally employed by acupuncturists and is based on the theory that there are five 'subtle elements': fire, earth, metal, water and wood. Any imbalance between the flow of energy from one element to the other will result in ill health. Diagnosis is made by examining the tone of voice, the colour tone of the face and the 'subtle smell' – not body odour – of the patient. It is also done by feeling twelve pulses – six on each wrist – which correspond to the twelve main 'meridians'. These are lines of subtle energy which run up or down the body, and each one corresponds to a major organ, such as the heart, stomach or liver. In acupuncture the main form of treatment is by inserting needles into specific acupuncture points which occur at intervals along each meridian. Incidentally the presence of these points can be verified with instruments which detect subtle changes in the electrical charge of the skin. Diagnosis is difficult enough for an expert; self-diagnosis is virtually impossible.

Muscle-testing (*Touch for Health*)

This involves testing the relative strengths of different muscles, mostly by using an arm or leg as a 'lever'. Muscle-testing existed for some years in hospital physiotherapy departments before it was ever applied to the natural therapies. Chiropractors in the USA first theorized, and then demonstrated, a connection between particular muscle tests and acupuncture meridians. To put it simply, muscle-testing can be used as a relatively simple form of oriental diagnosis – it helps to indicate which of the major organs are 'weak'. It is much easier to learn than oriental diagnosis, but even then it takes several weeks just to master the basic techniques. Touch for health is used by many body-treatment therapists, including some aromatherapists. While self-diagnosis is quite impossible, this is a technique which is taught to lay people.

Foot Reflexology

Also known as foot-zone therapy, this can be used purely for diagnosis or for treatment as well. It is based on the theory that the whole body is reflected in the feet – mainly in the soles, but also in the upper areas. The left half of the body shows up on the left foot, and the right half on the right foot. The feet are gently prodded with a thumb or finger all over, starting at the toes. Any areas which cause needle-like pain or an uncomfortable ache will correspond to the now familiar concept of 'weak areas' in the body. However, reflexology does tend to reveal more of a *physical* weakness, or at least 'unusual congestion', in the corresponding part, rather than what we would normally call a subtle energy weakness.

This method is often used by aromatherapists for diagnosis and sometimes for treatment too. It has to be said that treatment, which consists of massaging the painful areas, is distinctly uncomfortable, although the benefits may well justify the discomfort. Self-diagnosis, and even treatment, is difficult but feasible with an appropriate chart. Again, this technique can be learned by non-therapists, but some training should be undertaken before attempting to use it.

Other Body Reflexes

We are beginning to see that there are many parts of the body which act as mirrors, reflecting the state of health of distant organs. As well as the pulses and feet, there are equally elaborate techniques which are based on careful analysis of the eye, the ear, the large intestine, the whole face and the spine. Perhaps our bodies even hold other secrets which we have yet to discover. Some of these techniques probably sound incredible until you have experienced for yourself how telling and accurate they can be.

The Individual Blend

After the verbal consultation and holistic analysis, and if the aromatherapist is satisfied that there is no reason why you should not undergo aromatherapy treatment, then the next stage in events is the mixing of your 'individual prescription'. This is a blend of essential oils in a vegetable oil base which is designed to work on physical, mental and subtle energy problems all at the same time. This is not as difficult as it sounds; the right blend of oils will act on all levels because it represents what you, the 'whole you', needs. However, there will be times when supplementary treatment, such as baths or inhalations, will also be required.

A Tisserand-trained aromatherapist will use muscle-testing to test out and confirm which essential oils are best for you. For example, a patient arrives with a minor urinary infection. On testing, the muscles corresponding to the kidneys are found to be very weak; this test involves pressing down in a very specific way on the patient's raised leg while they are lying face up. Usually the patient is not at all surprised that the leg gives way in this situation. However, when the patient holds a bottle of sandalwood oil to the side of his or her face the leg tests strong – it does not move when pushed. This indicates that sandalwood oil is somehow strengthening a weakness a related to the kidneys. Even if you do not believe in the connection between muscle and organ there is no doubt that something positive is happening. It is not meant to be, but this kind of testing does seem like some kind of magic, and the patient, often surprised that their leg is now 'strong', can see and feel with their own body that a positive reaction has taken place, even before treatment has begun. This is also used as a measure of progress. If the patient returns a week later and the muscle test proves to be strong even without any essential oils then both therapist and patient can see that a real improvement has taken place. In our example, if the sandalwood oil had not had a positive effect then another oil would be tried, perhaps rose, juniper or tea-tree, until one is found that does work.

Other aromatherapists will use different esoteric techniques in selecting essential oils, like dowsing. This involves using the swing of a pendulum to indicate the most appropriate oils. Some therapists feel that they can rely entirely on their intuition, although the problem here is that intuition is sometimes quite wrong, and, if the therapist is having an off-day, the intuitive faculty is not going to be at its best. All of these techniques, including muscle-testing, need to be used in the context of a very sound practical knowledge of aromatherapy. They should never be used as a substitute for it.

Some aromatherapists will ask the patient which oil is preferred out of a small selection of oils. The importance of the patient liking the odour of an oil was half-recognized by Dioscorides 2000 years ago and it actually makes a lot of sense. I have found from experience that tastes in smell vary considerably. While most people adore jasmine, there are those who dislike it, and while many dislike patchouli it sends others into raptures. Nobody knows the reason for our individual preferences, but our noses could be telling us what is good for us and what is not. There is a danger that this idea could be taken too far, and it is not a practice I employ very often. Occasionally, if I am unsure which of two oils to use in a blend, I will ask the patient's opinion. If you positively dislike the oils your therapist has chosen for you do say so – the therapist may make a change, or may not, but say anyway. One more thing – do not expect your blend of oils to smell like commercial perfume because it will not. Natural oils have a different type of odour from commercial fragrances.

Some General Remarks

Sometimes patients are surprised by the amount of tension in their bodies. These tension areas are caused by many things, including posture, sport, gardening, even things like sewing. They can also be caused by mental and emotional tensions, especially repressed emotions. Massaging these tensions helps to release the emotional cause, by a reflex effect. After your treatment you will feel different, even if only slightly. Some people feel a little disorientated, or light-headed, or simply more energetic and relaxed. The release of toxins and of neurochemicals into the bloodstream is responsible for most of these feelings. Sometimes you may go through a short reaction period, during which time you feel worse – this has already been discussed. You should certainly feel better in some way within two days of your treatment.

Aromatherapy sessions normally last for an hour, although your first visit may be longer because of the consultation. Treatments are given weekly in the beginning and at some point are usually spaced out to once every two weeks and then once a month. Some patients like to keep coming indefinitely, once a month or once every three months, for maintenance treatments – these may be necessary in some cases to keep a condition at bay, especially if it was originally a long-standing problem. How long you would need to go for treatment is an impossible question to answer because it depends on so many things. It could be anything from three weeks to three years. Even if there is nothing much wrong with you (I have never met a perfectly healthy person) aromatherapy is a wonderful way of relaxing and improving, or maintaining, your health at the same time. Aromatherapists are experts at dealing with those minor problems which your general practitioner does not want to be bothered with and yet which could, in time, develop into something more serious.

CHAPTER SEVEN

ESSENTIAL OILS

To Make an Essence of any Herb

Take the foregoing water, and distill it in a gourd Glass . . . and there will come forth a Water and an Oil. The Oil separate from the Water, and keep it by it self . . . And by this means you shall have a most subtill essence, which being held over a gentle heat will fly up into the Glass and represent the perfect Idea of that Vegetable [Plant] whereof it is the essence.

The Art of Distillation, John French, 1651

Essential oils are products of nature. They are not in fact essential to plant life, but are found in all fragrant flowers and herbs. About 20 per cent of all medicinal herbs owe their healing properties to essential oils. They give fragrance to roses and lavender, and flavour to nutmeg and cinnamon. Many plants contain essential oils which are not commercially extracted, including flowers such as lilac, gardenia, lily of the valley and sweet pea. If you ever see 'essential oil of gardenia' you can be sure it is nothing but a synthetic perfume. Some exotic flower oils do exist, such as narcissus, tuberose, cassie and hyacinth, but these and others like them are all extremely expensive and it is unlikely that you will ever find them in a high-street shop. Prices would have to be in the region of £75 for a 10 ml bottle.

There are about 200 essential oils produced commercially in the world today, and some 50–100 of these are utilized in aromatherapy. They come from all parts of the globe, and from every conceivable plant part (see Table 3). Most of

Table 3. The fifty most commonly used essential oils in aromatherapy, and where they come from

Oil	Source	Country
Angelica	Roots	Germany
Basil	Herb	Italy
Bergamot	Fruit rind	Italy
Black Pepper	Fruit	India
Cajuput	Leaves of tree	Australia
Camphor	Wood	Japan
Cardamom	Seeds	India
Cedarwood	Wood	USA
Camomile (German)	Flowers	Germany
Camomile (Roman)	Flowers	Hungary
Cinnamon	Leaves	Sri Lanka
Clary Sage	Herb	France
Coriander	Seeds	USSR
Cypress	Leaves of tree	France
Clove	Flower buds	Madagascar
Eucalyptus	Leaves of tree	Spain
Fennel	Seeds	Italy
Frankincense	Gum from tree	Somalia
Galbanum	Gum from tree	Iran
Geranium	Leaves	Egypt
Ginger	Roots	India
Grapefruit	Fruit rind	USA
Hyssop	Herb	France
Jasmine	Flowers	Morocco
Juniper	Fruit	Yugoslavia
Immortelle	Flowers	Italy
Lavender	Flowers	France
Lemon	Fruit rind	Brazil
Lemongrass	Grass	China
Marjoram	Herb	Hungary
Melissa	Herb	France
Myrrh	Gum from tree	Somalia
Orange	Fruit rind	Brazil
Orange Blossom	Flowers	Tunisia
Patchouli	Leaves	Indonesia
Peppermint	Herb	USA
Petitgrain	Leaves of tree	Paraguay
Pine	Wood	USSR
Rose	Flowers	Bulgaria
Rosemary	Herb	Spain
Rosewood	Wood	Brazil
Sage	Herb	Yugoslavia
Sandalwood	Wood	India
Tea-tree	Leaves of tree	Australia

Table 3.—Cont.

Thyme	Herb	Spain
Verbena	Leaves	Algeria
Vetiver	Roots	Réunion
Yarrow	Flowers	Germany
Ylang-Ylang	Flowers	Madagascar
Violet	Leaves	Egypt

these are distilled in their country of origin. In the case of a fragile plant structure, such as a flower, the essential oil evaporates very readily and so is quite easily perceptible to the nose. It also has to be distilled very soon after harvesting, and some essential oils are still extracted by fairly primitive stills to be found among the fields where the plant is grown. In the case of a more solid plant structure, such as a bark, root or seed, the oil does not evaporate so readily and is less obvious to the nose. These plant materials do not have to be promptly distilled and in fact may be exported as raw materials for extraction in another country or simply stored for extraction at a later date. Large quantities of vetiver roots from Haiti or Réunion and iris roots from Italy are distilled in the South of France. This causes some confusion as to whether the essential oil is actually French or not. Iris root oil, known as orris root 'concrete' or iris butter, is not used in aromatherapy. Apart from its great expense it is unique in that the essential oil is actually quite solid, and it does not lend itself to dilution in vegetable oil.

The essential oil in a plant is present in tiny sacs, or globules. In some of the flat leaves, like eucalyptus or orange leaf, these sacs can be seen by holding the leaf up to a strong light source. This appearance of tiny blobs gave rise to the French name for orange leaf oil – *petitgrain*, meaning 'little bit'. The extraction of most essential oils is carried out by means of distillation, but the citrus oils –

bergamot, orange, grapefruit, etc. are extracted simply by pressing, or expression. Hard materials, such as gums, roots or woods, have to be chipped, or even powdered prior to distillation. The plant material, which will either be freshly harvested, or dry, is loaded into the still, which is in effect a giant pressure cooker (see Figure 12). Steam is passed, under

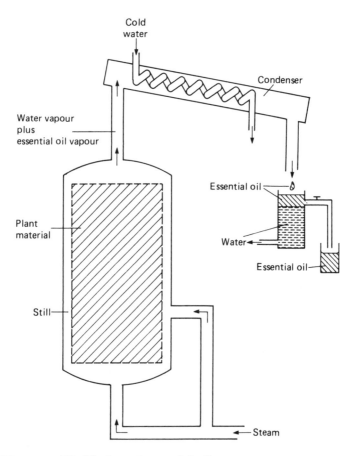

Figure 12. Distillation of essential oils.

pressure, through the plant material, and the heat causes the globules of essential oil in the plant to burst open, and the oil quickly evaporates. The steam, or water vapour, and the essential oil vapour then pass out from the top of the still and along a pipe which is water-cooled. This condenses the vapours back into liquids. It is then an easy matter to separate the water from the essential oil, since they do not mix, and the essence naturally floats on top of the water.

The average yield of essential oil from raw material is 1.5 per cent, which means that about 70 kg of plant material is required to produce 1 kg of essential oil. In some cases the yield is much higher. Frankincense gum, for instance, yields between 5 and 10 per cent, whereas rose petals only yield 0·015 per cent, so over 6000 kg of rose petals are required to obtain 1 kg of oil. It has been calculated that no less than *eight million* jasmine flowers go into each kilogram of jasmine oil. Rose and jasmine are, not surprisingly, the most expensive of all essences, and cost about fifty times more than most other oils.

Essential oils are all odorous and highly volatile, which means that they readily evaporate if given the opportunity. They are not greasy, are quite different from fatty oils, and have a consistency much more like water than oil. They will dissolve in pure alcohol, but not spirits, which never contain more than 50 per cent alcohol. They do not dissolve in water, but they do dissolve in all fats, oils and waxes, whether of animal, vegetable or mineral origin. So they will readily mix with vegetable oils, such as olive, almond, soya and so on, and also with beeswax and vaseline.

Essential oils are adversely affected by *light*, *heat*, *oxygen* and *moisture*. They should always be kept in dark bottles, away from heat or strong sunlight. They do not mind cold, but if kept in a refrigerator some of them will thicken and so will not pour very easily until they have been warmed. If kept under favourable conditions essential oils will last for at least one year, and some will last for five years or longer. However, there is a small group of oils which do tend to 'go off' after about six months. These are all the citrus oils – e.g. orange, lemon, and grapefruit – except for bergamot, which does keep well.

Below are listed some points to look out for when you are buying essential oils:

* Price is a good indication of quality. If the product is very cheap, it is probably also below par. On the other hand, if it is *very* much more expensive than average you may be paying more than you need to.
* Buy from a well-known, reputable supplier, preferably one who specializes in essential oils.
* The bottle. This should always be made of opaque glass, whether brown, blue, or some other colour. The neck of the bottle should incorporate a drop-dispenser, so that one drop at a time can be dispensed.
* Whenever possible buy undiluted oils. Some companies dilute their oils without any indication that they have done so. Some of the very costly oils are sold diluted to make them affordable. However, diluted oils are not suitable for most purposes, such as compresses, douches and inhalations, and in calculating number of drops.

It is important that only pure, good quality essential oils are used in aromatherapy. In recent years there has been some confusion between pure essential oils and so-called 'fragrance oils' or 'aromatic oils' which may be nothing more than diluted perfumes. Human nature being what it is there will always be those who attempt to pass off synthetic perfumes as being 'natural'. The usual excuse is that they do not contain any animal-derived ingredients, coupled with a homely, 'natural' packaging and company image – a clever seduction. At the time of writing the number of truly natural perfumes on the market is very close to zero, and this situation is unlikely to change. Pure essential oils are too expensive and simply do not provide the great range of fragrances which modern perfumery depends upon.

Originally perfumes consisted entirely of natural ingredients, for the simple reason that there was no alternative. About 150 years ago the average perfume was 85 per cent natural and 15 per cent synthetic. Since that time there has been a steady trend away from naturals and towards synthetics, and the figures are now completely reversed: the average modern perfume is 85 per cent synthetic and only 15 per cent natural. Here is a formula for a simple rose perfume, *Rose Fleurs*, from a classic French work on perfumery in 1931 by a certain Felix Cola:[1]

Rhodinol pure	50 grammes
Phenylethyl alcohol	10g
Ionone alpha	15g
Bulgarian rose *otto*	10g
Geraniol	10g
Rhodinyl acetate	5g
	100g

The only natural ingredient here is Bulgarian rose *otto*, and it comprises 10 per cent of the formula, a percentage which would be quite impossible in a modern perfume, because of cost. The perfume compound of an expensive, modern fragrance might contain something like 1 per cent of natural rose oil. The only reason that very costly natural oils like rose and jasmine are still produced commercially is that they cannot be successfully imitated or copied in the laboratory. Natural rose oil is composed of some 500 constituents, 490 of them at a level of less than 1 per cent. So far, in spite of knowing in some detail what rose oil is composed of, perfume chemists have been unable to copy it successfully. Combining the same chemicals in the same proportions simply does not work – the resulting liquid does not smell like the real thing. Obviously nature holds a few mysteries yet.

Although man-made ingredients constitute the majority of flavours and fragrances today, the essential oil industry is still a very big one. For instance, the annual world production of peppermint oil is 4·5 tonnes, or 4·5 million kg. Most of it is grown and produced in the USA, and goes into flavours for chewing-gum, mints and other confections and flavours. The world production of rose *otto* is only about 3000 kg, most of which goes into fragrances, although the demand for aromatherapy is beginning to affect the rose *otto* market. The production of rose *otto* is 1500 times less than that of peppermint, but because the price of rose is so much higher the total revenue is only ten times less. Eucalyptus oil, most of which now comes from Spain and Portugal, not Australia, is primarily used for pharmaceutical purposes.

Figure 13 illustrates the probable breakdown of essential oil usage worldwide. This breakdown is an estimate based on information provided by certain essential oil wholesalers and suppliers to the aromatherapy trade. The 2 per cent figure for aromatherapy does not apply to *all* essential oils, only to those commonly used in aromatherapy. However, since these include many of the relatively expensive oils, I think the figure can be taken as being reasonably accurate in monetary terms, if not in terms of volume. I would say that the percentage for aromatherapy ten years ago was about ten times less, 0·2 per cent. In five years from now it could be as high as 10 per cent.

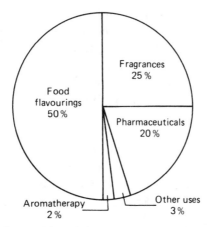

Figure 13. Estimated breakdown of essential oil usage.

A pure essential oil is a vibrant, dynamic liquid which almost seems to have a life quality of its own. An essential oil destined for aromatherapy should come from an organically grown, properly tended plant source, and certain standards are also required during distillation. This is the ideal, not the reality. However, as aromatherapy grows in popularity and usage so its needs are beginning to make themselves felt on the essential oil industry. A number of growers, distillers and even wholesalers are now conscious of the need for essential oils which are pure, handled with care and are produced only from the correct plant source.

Oils from organically grown plants are especially difficult to obtain in some cases, especially the citrus oils, and claims from suppliers that 'all our essential oils are organically grown' should be treated with a healthy degree of scepticism. Many of the oils have always been organically grown anyway, such as lavender, tea-tree and frankincense, but citrus trees are difficult to grow without some spraying. The new aromatherapy market is not so interested in fragrance or flavour, but in purity. As the demand from the perfumery industry continues its long-term march away from naturals (in spite of a recent reversal of this trend), so the medicinal usage of essential oils will continue to increase. In some cases, tea-tree oil for instance, the pharmaceutical industry will probably give impetus to this trend by adopting some of the essential oils and using them in commercial preparations.

There follows an outline of eight of the best-known essential oils. Since this is not an aromatherapy textbook I have not tried to give a detailed account of each oil and its healing properties. Much of the content is there purely for interest's sake, and I have included one or two amusing anecdotes. The section on tea-tree oil is an exception. Since it has come to the attention of aromatherapists in Europe only recently, it has not previously been written about in books on aromatherapy. As it also turns out to be one of the most useful essential oils I have taken this opportunity to describe its therapeutic action in some detail.

Clary Sage

Botanical name: *Salvia sclarea*   Family: *Labiatae*
Essence from: Herb and flowers   Cultivated in: France
Odour: Herbaceous and floral
Most common uses: Depression
                  Frigidity
                  Period pains
                  Pre-menstrual syndrome
                  Throat infections

Clary sage is botanically related to common sage, but the two essential oils are quite different and should not be

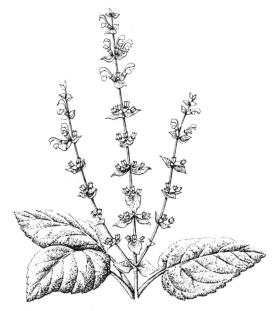

Figure 14. Clary sage (*Salvia sclarea*).

confused.* It does grow in England, and is widely cultivated for its essential oil in southern regions of Russia, but the Russian oil is inferior to the French. The name is believed to be a distortion of the common 'clear-eye', since a mucilage from the seeds was used to remove foreign particles from the eye.

The plant was well known in ancient times and has a tradition of medicinal use. In Tudor times the leaves were dipped in batter and fried to be served up with meat or omelettes. They were also used in scent bags and in *potpourri* and were added to fruit jellies. According to one source, in Jamaica clary sage leaves were boiled in coconut oil to make a remedy for scorpion stings.

* Common sage oil is moderately toxic and is not suitable for home use.

In Germany this plant is known as *muskateller salbei* or muscatel sage. It has been used for centuries by German wine merchants, who add it to Rheinish wine, giving it the flavour of muscatel wine. According to one author (1822) it has also been used in the past by English beer-makers for 'sophisticating beer, communicating considerable bitterness and intoxicating property, which produced an effect of insane exhilaration of spirits, succeeded by severe headache', while a seventeenth-century author writes: 'Some brewers of Ale and Beere doe put it into their drinke to make it more heady, fit to please drunkards, who thereby, according to their several dispositions, become either dead drunke, or foolish drunke, or madde drunke.'[2]

Clary sage is certainly one of the most effective euphoric essential oils, and of all the oils I know has the most drug-like effect. However, smelling the oil for a few moments is not sufficient, it must be evaporated into the air or used in massage. The first time I used the oil was when giving a massage, and both I and the patient became rather intoxicated. However, my experience pales beside that of Gordon Haddock, an aromatherapist, who wrote to me saying:

You asked for any results of treatments with essential oils. The most dramatic was a treatment I gave with clary sage oil. It was the first time I had used the oil and consequently have not used it since.

My patient was suffering from acute depression. During the treatment he became convinced he was floating in the air and kept opening his eyes, fearing he was about to bang his head on the ceiling! I barely finished the massage when I had to crawl off to the nearest empty floor space where I 'passed out'.

I came to an hour later and woke my patient with some coffee. The treatment was totally successful, and he left somewhat high and ethereal. When I work out some form of mask to wear I might consider using it again!

I wrote back to Mr Haddock, wondering if he had perhaps been exaggerating a little, and received a reply from the patient, which included the following comments: 'I am able to confirm that the results were truly overwhelming ... At the completion of the one hour massage we both dozed for an hour, drifting in and out of a hazy mist of herbal influence. The strong effects lasted for three hours after the completion of the massage.' I have included these accounts because they graphically illustrate the euphoric effects of aromatherapy – much better than I could in my own words. Let me assure you, however, that imagined levitation, and the very strong narcotic effects described here, are quite unusual. Clary sage is undoubtedly one of the most effective essential oils for treating depression of all kinds.

Clary sage is also thought to be an aphrodisiac. According to Rovesti: 'The musky odour of the flowers and of the essential oil justifies their very effective erogenous application.' No doubt the euphoric and aphrodisiac qualities are linked in some way. There is some suspicion that it might stimulate the release of adrenaline, and it certainly has some effect on the sex hormones, probably stimulating the release of oestrogen. This links up, not only with its aphrodisiac quality, but with its very useful application in many types of menstrual disorder, including the most common, period pains and pre-menstrual syndrome. In the case of the latter its euphoric properties are also of great value. Clary sage oil is sedative, and reduces high blood pressure.[3]

Lavender

Botanical name: *Lavandula officinalis*   Family: *Labiatae*
Essence from: Flowering tops   Cultivated in: France, Tasmania

Odour: Herbaceous and floral

Most common uses: Bites and stings
     Burns
     Eczema /dermatitis
     Insomnia
     Nervous tension (anxiety)
     Lice
     Asthma
     Immune deficiency (persistent in-
      fections)

The lavender plant was probably introduced to England by the Romans, who often used it in connection with bathing. Its name derives from the Latin *lavare*, meaning 'to wash'. The ancient Greeks, Romans and Persians all burned

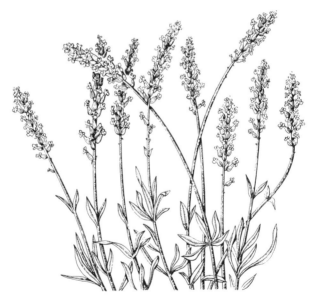

Figure 15. Lavender (*Lavandula officinalis*).

lavender in sick rooms and to fumigate their houses against epidemics. It was also used in this way during the European plagues. As early as 1694 John Pechey spoke of using the essential oil for head lice: 'The oyl of it kills Lice in Childrens Heads, their Heads being anointed with it.'

Lavender is one of the mildest, and yet most effective, of all essential oils. No home should be without it. Burns, headaches, indigestion, insect bites and stings, infections, insomnia, sores, eczema – all of these common complaints yield to the gentle healing powers of this wonderful oil. It is antiseptic, gently relaxing, slightly analgesic and very healing.[2] The image of lavender water and ladies of a certain age persists to this day. Indeed it was one of the most popular fragrances in the seventeenth and eighteenth centuries, and ladies would literally douse themselves with it to protect against foul smells and fainting. To quote John Gerarde, 1633: 'The distilled water of Lavender smelt unto, or the temples and forehead bathed therewith, is a refreshing to them that have the Catalepsy, a light migram [migraine], and to them that use to swoune much.' Strange how 'swouning' has gone out of fashion, and lavender water along with it. If anything, I suppose, swooning has been replaced by headaches. No matter, lavender will help in either case, and it can sometimes be of use in migraines, as was noticed by Gerarde, and also by a certain lady from Birmingham:

My sister suffers periodically from 'tension' migraine. A few days ago she had what she thought was going to be a bad attack. I gave her three drops of lavender oil to take on a lump of brown sugar. In a matter of minutes, to her great surprise and delight, the eye symptoms disappeared. A little later the headache was gone also. She felt tired for the rest of the day, as she usually does after a migraine, but she was very pleased indeed to have recovered so well and so quickly.

Please note that lavender oil on its own should not be regarded as a cure for migraine, but sometimes it does bring considerable relief.

The effectiveness of lavender oil on burns is perhaps the most dramatic and telling phenomenon in aromatherapy. It has to be experienced to be believed. Valnet writes:

A colleague of mine, not a man to waste time when it comes to forming an opinion about the curative properties of a given substance, once went ahead and deliberately burned two fingers on his left hand. He immediately treated one finger with the mixture of aromatic essences. The other he left alone. In a matter of minutes there was no pain in the treated finger, and the next day not even a sign of the burn. The other finger, however, was very sore and covered in blisters, giving him ample time to observe and feel the difference . . .[4]

The mixture referred to is based on oils of lavender, geranium, thyme, rosemary and sage. Generally I have found lavender to be the most effective. In *The Art of Aromatherapy* I give an account of a serious steam burn treated with lavender oil. Again the results were dramatic. Just part of the effectiveness of lavender is due to its apparent ability to stimulate the healing process, so that the formation of new, healthy skin is actually speeded up. There is a correlation here with the stimulation of the immune response – stimulating both the production and the activity of certain types of white blood cell. When needed, lavender appears to be capable of stimulating cellular growth, and in this sense could be regarded as rejuvenating.

More than once I have been asked if lavender oil could aggravate, or even cause, leukaemia, since it stimulates the production of white blood cells. The simple answer is no. In fact the essential problem in leukaemia is the failure of white blood cells to mature. As the disease progresses these quite useless cells replace the normal, healthy ones. If anything, lavender would help the condition by stimulating the growth of normal cells. In 1935 a certain Monsieur Godissart took aromatherapy to Los Angeles. Apparently this man composed a product, which he called *Vita-Cell*, in which French lavender oil played a significant role.[5] It is claimed that this product was used to successfully treat certain types of skin cancer, and before and after photographs of skin cancers treated by this man, who obviously understood the cell-vitalizing nature of lavender, give evidence for this. If lavender oil was a synthetic chemical it probably would stimulate cell growth regardless of circumstances, but natural oils seem, with few exceptions, only to work in harmony with the body, always helping it to regain its normal state of balance. While there is a possibility that lavender oil may be of use in treating certain cancers, there is absolutely no proof of this, and I am not suggesting that anyone, medical or otherwise, should use lavender oil in this way.

Godissart makes another dramatic claim, this time with no supportive evidence, that: 'The bite of the black widow spider, until now considered to be mortal, is rendered harmless, thanks to the antitoxic power of lavender.' Perhaps it is true, perhaps not, I certainly have no plans to try out this particular claim. However, there is no doubt that lavender does work on many types of insect bites and stings, and it does seem to have the power to neutralize the toxins involved. I have experienced this many times myself, and I know of dozens of others who have found the same. Bee stings, wasp stings, gnat bites, mosquito bites and nettle stings, at least from the species we have in England, are all neutralized by lavender oil applied neat to the bite or sting. Although it does not repel insects, lavender is very useful to take with you if you are travelling to warmer climes.

Peppermint

Botanical name: *Mentha piperita*   Family: *Labiatae*
Essence from: Leaves   Cultivated in: USA, Brazil, Europe
Odour type: Minty
Most common uses: Nausea
        Indigestion
        Colic
        Diarrhoea
        Flatulence
        Headache
        Pain
        Mental fatigue
        Influenza
        Colds
        Sinus congestion

According to Greek mythology the god Pluto found himself attracted to the young nymph, Mentha. Pluto's infuriated wife, Persephone, pursued Mentha and trod her ferociously into the ground. Pluto then changed Mentha into a delightful herb. The herb has been used for centuries as a medicine, especially for its peerless healing effect in digestive problems. The herb owes its therapeutic properties entirely to its essential oil, whose fragrance is dominated by a constituent called *menthol*. Menthol constitutes about one-third of the essential oil, is a clear, solid crystal in its pure form and is often used in liniments, inhalants and strong mints. Peppermint herb is grown extensively in the USA and is the number three essential oil in terms of quantity. Currently some 4·5 million kg are produced worldwide per annum. This is mainly to provide for the huge demand in the flavouring industry. Peppermint oil is used extensively in toothpastes, chewing-gums, mints, chocolates, breath

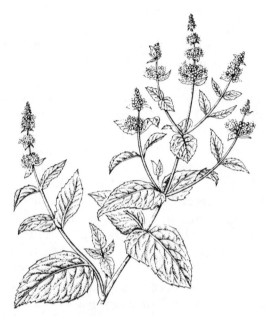

Figure 16. Peppermint (*Mentha piperita*).

fresheners, 'menthol' cigarettes and so on, but is hardly used at all in perfumery. Menthol (either extracted from natural sources, or synthetic) is often used to reinforce the cooling effect of the oil, which is the main reason for its use. However, menthol is rarely used on its own, because its flavour is very much inferior to that of the natural oil. The good news is that the great majority of peppermint flavours are natural, and there are no signs that this is likely to change.

Peppermint oil is the remedy *par excellence* for digestive disorders and makes a wonderfully safe and effective home remedy, although some care needs to be exercised if using it on the skin. It relieves nausea, indigestion and colic, prevents flatulence and bloating, and is an excellent first-aid remedy for diarrhoea. It will also help to prevent travel sickness and morning sickness. It stimulates the digestive process and is a very good intestinal antiseptic. In November 1979 the doctor's column in a national Sunday newspaper extolled the virtues of peppermint oil for a condition known as irritable bowel syndrome (IBS), a very common problem.[6] The doctor explained that the effectiveness of the oil was partly due to its antispasmodic properties – it relaxes the intestinal muscle, if it is in spasm. He also mentioned a double-blind trial in which people suffering from recurrent colic attacks were given peppermint oil capsules. These all looked and smelt the same, but only some of the patients were taking natural peppermint oil. Only the real thing gave continued relief. He also stated that he prefers giving peppermint oil to sedatives or increased fibre in the diet. (It is worth noting here that IBS is often related to an allergy to certain foods.) In September 1980 a European patent was filed for a medicine to treat 'irritable colon syndrome, and for relief of gastric discomfort and of flatulent colic'. The medicine is based on essential oils, in particular peppermint, and a trial is quoted in which thirty-two patients with IBS were given capsules containing two and a half drops of peppermint oil to take three times a day before meals. Of the thirty-two, twenty-five were reported to show a good or excellent response. One could speculate that the other seven might respond to another essential oil or that they are highly allergic to something they are eating.

Peppermint oil does have anti-inflammatory properties, but great care is needed in diluting it sufficiently, otherwise it will have the opposite effect to the one desired. It is also a mild analgesic and will sometimes relieve headaches or nerve pains. When inhaled or tasted the menthol in the oil has a noticeably cooling effect, and it is well known that it also has a slight numbing action on the trigeminal nerve, which travels across the cheek. Small amounts of peppermint are said to be stimulating, and large amounts to be sedative. It is certainly one of the brain-stimulating essential oils and will, at least for short periods, aid concentration and memory. It is also of great value in inhalations for colds, flu and sinus congestion, although too much can be too strong and will irritate the nose. For inhalations or internal use, one, two or three drops is quite sufficient. Suggestion – try using peppermint oil as a natural alternative to aspirin.

Rose

Botanical name: *Rosa damascena*   Family: *Rosaceae*
Essence from: Flowers   Cultivated in: Bulgaria, Turkey, Morocco
Odour type: Floral
Most common uses: Anxiety
                    Constipation
                    Depression
                    Many emotional problems
                    Gall bladder problems
                    Hangover
                    Menstrual disorders
                    Pre-menstrual syndrome
                    Sexual dysfunction (impotence/frigidity)
                    Skin care (sensitive or ageing skin)

It is unfortunate that rose oil is extremely expensive, because I rate it among the three most useful essential oils, along with lavender and tea-tree. There are two quite different extracts from roses – the essential oil, also known as rose *otto*, and colourless, and the absolute, which has an orange colour. The absolute is cheaper, although still very pricey, and is the one usually sold as 'rose oil'; however, the essential oil is very much more effective in aromatherapy, and it is this, not the absolute, which I am describing here.

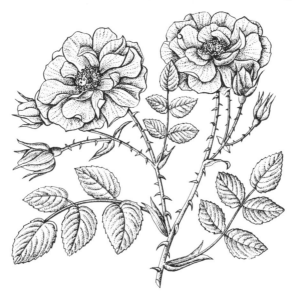

Figure 17. Rose (*Rosa damascena*).

The main reason for its expense is the very low yield of essential oil from the roses; at 0·015 per cent it is exactly *100 times* less than the average yield for essential oils. When we consider this, the fact that it is fifty times more costly than most other oils seems quite reasonable. Its price puts it out of reach to the average consumer, but it is invaluable to both the aromatherapist and the master perfumer.

The rose is surely the most written about, the most loved, the most praised and the most sought-after fragrance of all flowers. The ancient Persians called it 'gul', or 'flower' –

in other words, *the* flower. The art of distilling roses originated in ancient Persia, although in those times the distillation *water* was actually more prized than the essential oil.
Between the years AD 810 and 817 the Province of Faristan
paid an annual tribute of 30,000 bottles of rose water to the
Treasury of Baghdad. Faristan also exported rose water to
China, India, Yemen, Egypt and Spain at that time. The
rose became a Persian symbol and was used to adorn the
shields of Persian warriors. Rose water was (and still is)
sprinkled over guests on their arrival as a sign of welcome.
It was taken as a drink, flavoured with sugar and cinnamon
and was used to flavour numerous other delicacies. Today,
virtually all rose-flavoured confections, rose perfumes and
even rose waters are flavoured or scented with a synthetic
rose substitute.

Rose water and rose oil were first distilled in Persia, and
the town of Shiraz, near the Persian Gulf, became the centre
of the industry. Kaempfer, in 1684, described rose oil
production on his visit to Persia: 'The roses of Shiraz are
remarkable for yielding on distillation a fatty matter like
butter, which is called *Aettr Gyl* [rose *otto*]. This substance
is more valuable than gold, and nothing in the world pos-
sesses a perfume so agreeable and sweet.' The seventeenth
century also saw the beginning of commercial rose oil
production in Bulgaria. The Bulgarians have an expression
which translates as 'as expensive as rose oil'. For many
years they have been the world's main producers, although
both Turkey and Morocco are now strong rivals, also
producing good quality oil from the damask rose. Bulgarian
rose oil comes from roses grown in one particular area in
the foot-hills of the Balkan mountains, near the town of
Kazanlik, in central Bulgaria. The roses bloom for just
thirty days, and are rapidly hand-picked in the morning
during July or August. As the sun rises the essential oil

content of the flowers drops sharply, due to evaporation, and there is little enough of it to begin with. An experienced picker can pick up to 50 kg per day, enough to yield a mere 7.5 ml of precious essence. The harvest must be processed within twenty-four hours, and the exhausted flowers are used to manure the rose fields or as fodder mixtures.

In China a different species, *Rosa rugosa*, has been used medicinally since early times. According to Shih-Chen the flowers are used 'in all diseases of the liver, to scatter abscesses, and in blood diseases generally'.[7] He writes that the essential oil of this same rose acts on 'the liver, stomach, and blood. It drives away melancholy.' Culpeper also mentions that red roses 'strengthen the liver', and in eighteenth-century Bulgaria the 'juice' of fresh roses was used in the treatment of jaundice. Modern research confirms its effect on the liver and gall bladder. In 1972 a Russian report concluded that rose oil increased the production and secretion of bile when it was fed to rats.[8] In Bulgaria it has been used to treat inflammation of the gall bladder and similar disorders. Since the liver is undoubtedly affected by alcohol, perhaps the ancient Romans were on to a good thing when they drank rose water to prevent hangover. I have found rose oil useful in treating the effects of alcoholism and have also found it useful in counteracting certain negative emotions – envy, jealousy, resentment – all of which are associated with the liver and gall bladder in traditional oriental medicine.

In Bulgaria, rose water is a traditional remedy for burns, and recent studies have shown rose oil to be both antihistaminic (anti-inflammatory) and antiseptic. Bulgarian researchers have found it useful in treating pulmonary abscesses and other lung diseases, and have also established that rose oil is a diuretic, a laxative, an oxyuricide (kills certain intestinal worms) and a mild local anaesthetic.[9]

Rosemary

Botanical name: *Rosmarinus officinalis*   Family: *Labiatae*

Essence from: Leaves   Cultivated in: Tunisia

Odour: Camphoraceous

Most common uses: Hair loss
    Mental fatigue
    Physical weakness
    Rheumatism
    Muscular aches
    Liver and gall bladder problems

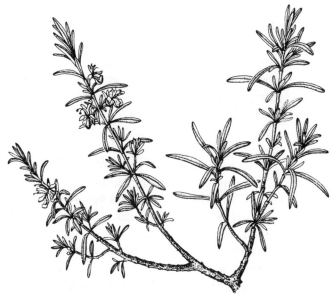

Figure 18. Rosemary (*Rosmarinus officinalis*).

Rosemary was the main ingredient of 'Hungary water', the first toilet water to make an impact in Europe, in 1370. A

U S advertisement of Hungary water in the 1920s stated: 'Now as it is certain that Rosemary has the power to increase the memory and invigorate the brain ... we cannot be surprised to learn that Orators, Clergymen, Lecturers, Authors, and Poets give it the preference.' In 1516 the *Grete Herbal* noted that rosemary was 'For weyknesse of ye brayne', and even Shakespeare had Ophelia comment: 'There's rosemary, that's for remembrance.' Were they all under a common delusion, perhaps blindly repeating what may have started as a whim, or does rosemary oil really stimulate the mental faculty and the memory?

In 1976 I treated an eleven-year-old boy whose mother brought him to see me because he was having a lot of difficulty in concentrating in class. This was not a long-term problem; his schoolwork had only begun to suffer during the past few months. After three treatments with diluted rosemary oil and a full spinal massage his schoolwork had improved noticeably and he was altogether brighter and more lively. He only had the three treatments, but two years later he was still going strong. This does not prove anything, but does add to the circumstantial evidence. We do know that rosemary is a nervous stimulant, and various different studies have shown that it stimulates heart action, respiration, digestion, kidney function, liver function, gall bladder function, blood circulation and the adrenal glands. It is in fact the most stimulating of all essential oils. If you should ever come across someone whose heart is failing, rub undiluted rosemary oil into their chest, right over the heart. It is harmless, and just might help save a life. You should also do everything else possible, of course.

We know that rosemary is a peerless stimulant, and since most of its stimulating effects take place via the nervous system it would not be surprising to learn that it stimulates the centre of nervous control – the brain itself. We also know that there are very close links in the brain between odour and memory, so I think it all adds up to confirm what was already known centuries ago. Of course they did not have the benefit of what we know now, but Conrad Gesner, writing in 1559, made a remarkably accurate observation when he said of rosemary: 'It strengtheneth the harte, the braine, the sinnewes [muscles] and the hoole bodye.' One could perhaps update this by claiming that 'rosemary refreshes the parts other oils cannot reach'.

Because of its stimulating effect on blood and lymph flow, especially when applied through the skin, rosemary oil is useful for all kinds of aches and pains, whether due to rheumatism, sprains, strains or simply overexertion of muscles.[2] It also stimulates the scalp, and it has been claimed that it will make hair grow on bald patches. This is not completely true, nor is it completely untrue. I have seen cases where it is has done just that, and yet it certainly does not work for everyone. Some years ago the London *Evening News* carried a report concerning a Woking beautician/aromatherapist who was causing something of a stir by 'curing baldness'. The first time it happened she was, apparently, massaging a lady's head to relieve her tension headaches. After three months of treatment new hair began to sprout on her head. The intrepid aromatherapist decided to test this out on fifty people, and had great success with many of them, including some who had tried every other preparation on the market. One, a local police officer, had been steadily getting balder since the age of eighteen. At forty-two his hair was now beginning to grow back, which the newspaper demonstrated with a photograph. The exact formula was not revealed, but the aromatherapist made it quite clear that she was using a blend of essential oils. While she did not mention rosemary oil, I have a very strong hunch that it played a significant role in her formula.

Sandalwood

Botanical name: *Santalum album*   Family: *Santalaceae*
Essence from: Wood   Cultivated in: India
Odour: Rich woody
Most common uses: Cystitis and urinary infections
Laryngitis
Throat infections
Skin care (dry skin)
Auto-immune deficiency (persistent infections)

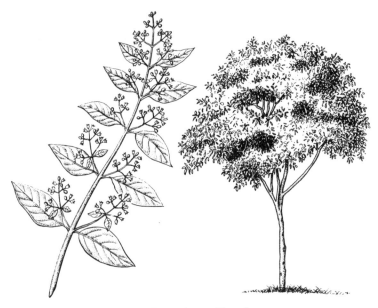

Figure 19. Sandalwood (*Santalum album*).

In China sandalwood is known as *chan-t'an*, which is an imitation of the Sanskrit *chandana*, the original Indian name. 'Tan' also means 'true' or 'sincere' and refers to the use of the wood as incense. In the Far East sandalwood incense is very widely used, although much of it contains little or no genuine sandalwood. It is sought after as the most prized incense to burn at funerals, and to remember the dead, especially in Japan, where ancestors are greatly revered. In China sandalwood incense is burned continuously under a portrait of the deceased until the funeral takes place. In India it is burned at funerals, and the wealthier the deceased, the more sandalwood is consumed. In 1984 the then prime minister of India, Indira Ghandi, was assassinated. Those who saw the televised funeral will remember an enormous funeral pyre, consisting largely of sandalwood, upon which her body was cremated.

Of all the aromatics sandalwood has the strongest tradition of religious use in the East, and is the equivalent of frankincense in Western religious ceremony. Hindu holy men use a sandalwood paste, coloured yellow and applied to the forehead, as a symbol of their spirituality. In Hindu marriages sandalwood is burned on the sacred fire in the 'marriage tent' so that its odorous fumes waft over the bridal couple. The Indians have also made use of its medicinal properties for the past 1000 years, and they long ago recognized its value in genito-urinary problems. Traditional uses in China include treating acne, hiccups and vomiting.

The Chinese mandarins traditionally burnt sandalwood incense as an offering to the Emperor to whom they came to pay homage. The demand led to its cultivation in the Lingnan region, which was successful for a while. However, the sandalwood is one of the slowest growing of all trees (they take about thirty years to reach twenty-five feet) and demand far outstripped supply. Few sandalwood trees now survive in China, and very little of the wood leaves India, but huge amounts of so-called 'sandalwood incense' are still consumed in the Far East.

The essential oil is quite well-known for its sweet, woody fragrance and, used alone, it makes a passable perfume. It is one of the most long-lasting of all essential oils, and is used in perfumes as a 'fixative'. It is one of the many relaxing oils and is often of use in treating stress-related problems. It is also a useful antiseptic, especially in urinary and throat infections. Rubbed diluted or undiluted into the neck area it will help a sore throat, and even helps in laryngitis.[2] One of the delegates at a public seminar I was giving in 1984 had laryngitis and could only speak in a whisper. Perhaps foolishly I claimed that I might be able to restore her voice and, in front of fifty people, rubbed some sandalwood oil into her neck. Two hours later her voice had returned to normal, much to the amazement of the other delegates, and much to my relief.

As well as being useful in specific infections, sandalwood is one of the oils which stimulate the immune system. Regular sandalwood baths, for instance, will help to keep your system resistant to infection. The oil is regarded by many as an aphrodisiac, and certainly has some effect in this area, although perhaps not as much as certain other oils. I think it could well be regarded as a sexual restorative. The oil is also very much used in skin care, especially for treating dry skin and acne.

Tea-tree

Botanical name: *Melaleuca alternifolia*
Family: *Myr   taceae*
Essence from: Leaves   Cultivated in: Australia
Odour: Spicy
Most common uses: almost any infection, including
> Respiratory
> Urinary
> Skin
> Vaginal
> Insect bites and stings
> Burns
> Cold sores
> Mouth ulcers
> Thrush
> Lice, ringworm and athlete's foot
> Boils

Tea-tree oil is comparable to lavender oil, not only in that it has similar uses, but also in that they both have so many possible applications that it is difficult to know where to start. Let us start at the beginning. For countless centuries the Bundjalung Aborigines used crushed tea-tree leaves as a poultice for infected wounds and skin problems. They inhabit the area where tea-trees are to be found, a relatively small, swampy region along the north coast of New South Wales. When Captain Cook visited the area his sailors brewed up tea-tree leaves to make a 'Spicey and refreshing tea', a welcome change from the monotony of their normal beverage. The name has stuck ever since. I think I should say at this point that some of the claims made for tea-tree oil may sound exaggerated – they are not. Tea-tree is one of the most thoroughly researched of all essential oils, and

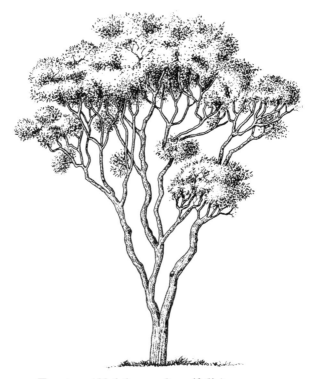

Figure 20. Tea-tree (*Melaleuca alternifolia*).

is surely the most generally useful as an antiseptic, and yet it has not previously been discussed at any length in books on aromatherapy.

In appearance tea-tree leaves are very like those of the cypress tree, and might be more accurately described as fronds. The myrtle family, to which this tree belongs, also includes some well-known aromatic trees, like myrtle, eucalyptus and clove. Of the well-known aromatics eucalyptus oil is the nearest in fragrance to that of tea-tree, which, however, has a more spicy, agreeable odour. The tree itself is rather like a trunk with a bush on top, and does not have the sleek form of cultivated cypress trees, but they are incredibly hardy and disease-resistant. For many years tea-trees were the bugbear of dairy farmers in the region, who found that nothing less than uprooting them would prevent them growing again. Its recuperative powers are astonishing; trees cut to within two feet of the ground, leaving nothing but a stump, are flourishing again with thick foliage within eighteen months.

The first to recognize the unique qualities of the essential oil was a government chemist from Sydney, A. R. Penfold. In 1925 he announced the results of laboratory experiments which showed that the oil was twelve times stronger than phenol (carbolic acid) which was then the universal standard for antiseptic substances. This led to further research and to the increasing use of the oil in medicine, dentistry and as a home remedy. In 1930 a report in the *Medical Journal of Australia*[10] commented on its non-toxicity and lack of irritancy. The report noted enthusiastically that tea-tree oil dissolved pus and left the surfaces of infected wounds clean so that its germicidal action became more effective and without any apparent damage to the tissues. 'Dirty wounds, such as are frequently seen as the result of street accidents, may be washed or syringed out with a 10% watery lotion; the solvent properties will loosen and bring away the dirt which is usually ground in . . . healing will readily take place.' In 1936 the same journal reported a very bad case of diabetic gangrene successfully treated with tea-tree oil. In 1937 it was pointed out that one of the outstanding features of the oil is that the presence of blood, pus or other organic matter actually *increases* the oil's antiseptic powers by some 10 to 12 per cent.[11]

During the Second World War tea-tree oil was issued in first aid kits to army and navy units in the tropical regions.

At one point demand so outstripped supply that synthetic antiseptics had to be substituted. This, coupled with the fervent post-war interest in antibiotic drugs, led to a decline of interest in tea-tree, which persisted right up to the 1970s. In April 1972 the results of a very thorough study were published on the use of tea-tree oil in many common foot problems.[12] The study covered sixty patients and concluded that the oil had relieved or eliminated foot symptoms in fifty-eight of them. Of these, results were graded as *excellent* in thirty-eight cases. The problems treated included athlete's foot, corns, callouses and bunions, hammer toes, skin peeling or cracking, fungal infection under toe-nails and bromhidrosis.* The study took place over a period of six years, and treatment times varied from three weeks to four years. In his conclusion the author, Morton Walker, observes that, overall, the best results were obtained in treating bromhidrosis, an 'unpleasant and embarrassing condition'. The athlete's foot cases were found to be caused by one or more of four fungi (including *Candida albicans*), all of which responded to tea-tree oil.

Ringworm is a condition closely related to athlete's foot, and almost as common. Both are caused by similar fungi. There have been a great many reports of ringworm being rapidly cleared up with tea-tree oil, and I have treated two cases, both of which were clear within three to four days. In June 1962 an American report was published in *Obstetrics and Gynecology* on the use of tea-tree oil in trichomonal vaginitis.[13] Vaginitis simply means vaginal inflammation, which in this case is caused by *Trichomonas*, a very tiny animal microbe, a flagellate creature, which is a common cause of greenish-yellow discharge, often foul smelling, and soreness in the area. The study comprised 130 women,

* Bromhidrosis is the medical term for 'smelly feet' and is caused by malodorous perspiration.

including ninety-six cases of trichomonal vaginitis, and also several cases of thrush and cervicitis. As controls the author, Dr Eduardo F. Peña, treated fifty other cases with standard antitrichomonal suppositories. The tea-tree oil was applied diluted by means of saturated tampons and douches, but was not given orally. Out of the 130 patients, all were successfully treated, and results were similar to the control group. Many patients commented on the pleasant odour of the oil, its cooling soothing effect and its efficiency in removing obnoxious vaginal odours. None of them complained of any irritation or burning.

More recently (1985) Dr Paul Belaiche conducted two studies featuring tea-tree oil, the first of these on twenty-eight cases of thrush (infestation of the vagina with *Candida albicans*).[14] *Candida albicans* is normally present in the vagina, but its growth is kept in check by certain bacteria. A common cause of thrush is antibiotic therapy which results in the beneficial bacteria being destroyed, thus allowing *Candida* to flourish. This results in a white discharge, often with itching, soreness and pain – a very common condition. For this study tea-tree oil was made into capsules for insertion into the vagina once every night. After the first week one patient felt vaginal burning, so discontinued treatment, but none of the others had any similar symptoms. After thirty days the twenty-seven patients were examined, and twenty-three showed a complete cure with no further discharge or burning. The other four showed a moderate improvement. Biological tests confirmed that twenty-one patients were clear of *Candida*. Belaiche observes that tea-tree oil is as effective as several other essential oils, but is notably less irritating: 'We have been happily astonished at the results obtained . . . the essential oil of *melaleuca* has entered the team of the major essential oils and emerges as an antiseptic and anti-fungal weapon of the first order in phyto-aroma-therapy.'

In Belaiche's second study with tea-tree oil, twenty-six female patients, with *chronic* cystitis were given the oil orally over a period of six months.[15] This was a double-blind trial, in which half the patients were given a placebo which had the odour of tea-tree. After six months none of the placebo group showed any improvement. Out of the thirteen who took tea-tree oil, seven were cured after six months, which, for such a chronic condition, is a significant result. As many have done before, Belaiche comments in his conclusion on the very low toxicity and irritancy of tea-tree oil.

Tea-tree oil has also been used successfully in the treatment of many other conditions, most of them either infectious conditions or skin conditions. It is now increasingly used by herbal practitioners in Australia, as it is by the layperson. Cuts, wounds, ulcers, sores, boils, burns, ringworm, athlete's foot, psoriasis, impetigo, nappy rash, anal and genital pruritis, cold sores, lice, urinary and vaginal infections, genital herpes, throat, bronchial and sinus infections, bad breath, mouth ulcers, infected gums and many other conditions have all responded remarkably well to treatment with this astonishing essential oil.

Like oils of lavender and peppermint, tea-tree is an ideal home remedy, and takes care of some of the most bothersome problems, whose nuisance value far outstrips their seriousness. It is even an effective remedy for leeches. Research has shown that the oil is four to five times stronger than the usual household disinfectants, and yet it is kinder to the skin, and of course is completely natural.[16] It is also relatively inexpensive and the problems it is used for are among the easiest to research. These combined facts have led to the prediction that demand for tea-tree oil will multiply some fifty times over the next few years and it is bound to feature in many natural remedies and patent medicines for home treatment.

Tea-tree oil should not be regarded as a cure-all, and will not work for everyone. However, it is one of the most exciting essential oils to emerge in recent years and, apart from its curative powers, is performing a valuable service in drawing attention to the antimicrobial powers of essential oils, and to the benefits of aromatherapy as a whole.

As an interesting conclusion, the following sheds some light on the antitoxic properties of tea-tree oil.

The venom toxicity of the black widow spider may be matched by that of the funnel web spider found only in New South Wales, Australia. This spider first made the news in 1927 when a two-year-old boy was bitten by one and died within ninety minutes. Since then five other deaths have been reported. The latest was a seventeen-year-old pregnant woman, who died in Sydney in 1970 after being bitten on the breast.

The following account dates from May 1983, and comes from Harry H. Bungwahl, New South Wales:

A rather extraordinary episode happened to me recently involving tea-tree oil. I was bitten on the foot by a funnel-web spider . . . It happened at night time about 1 a.m. He gave me a vicious bite, and it was very painful . . . I lay down on the bed and tried to think of some way to soothe the pain of the bite, which was very severe. I then thought of the small bottle of tea-tree oil which was in the bathroom. My wife went and got it and applied some to the bite and there was an immediate easing of the pain. My wife then went to ring up Taree Hospital, and while she was doing that I put some more tea-tree oil onto the bite which, in a short time, stopped being painful! My son drove me to the Taree Hospital – the foot was no longer painful but my lips and fingers were still tingling . . . the spider was identified as a male funnel-web spider all right . . . I was given no treatment but was kept under observation for a period of four hours, and then discharged.

It is interesting that both tea-tree oil and the funnel web spider are found only in New South Wales.

Ylang-ylang

Botanical name: *Cananga odorata*   Family: *Anonaceae*
Essence from: Flowers   Cultivated in: Madagascar
Odour type: Heady floral
Most common uses: Depression
　　　　　　　　　　Impotence
　　　　　　　　　　Frigidity

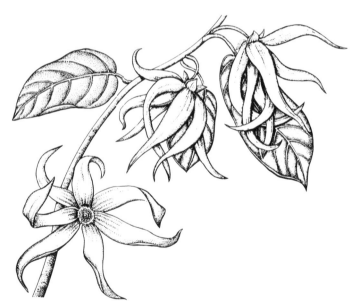

Figure 21. Ylang-ylang (*Cananga odorata*).

Although it does affect the physical body, ylang-ylang is one of the most emotionally evocative essential oils, and its use in aromatherapy is principally on this level. The ylang-ylang plant is a tree which grows in Indonesia and the Philippines (the name is Malay, and means 'flower of flowers'), although most of the commercial plantations are now in Madagascar. The tree grows to a height of up to twenty-five feet, and the unusually shaped yellow flowers are picked in the early morning for distillation. The odour is intensely sweet and heady, almost creamy, and not liked by everyone in concentration. One warning about ylang-ylang oil; if you use too much, or smell it for too long undiluted, it can give you a headache. In dilution, or mixed with other oils, most people find the scent irresistible. It is widely used in perfumery, especially in floral and oriental-type perfumes, and is the main ingredient of the old 'Macassar oil'. It is also used in a number of food flavours, including some ice-creams.

In 1866 Guibourt reported in his *Natural History of Simple Drugs* that ylang-ylang flowers were made into a pomade with coconut oil in the Molucca islands. In the winter this was rubbed into the whole body to guard against fevers, and it was used all year round by young women to perfume their hair after bathing. Philippino and Malayan girls decorate their hair with a single flower. Although chemically they are quite different, the fragrance of ylang-ylang has often been compared to that of jasmine, a much more costly essence. Of the many reputed aromatic aphrodisiacs ylang-ylang and jasmine are probably the most reliable. In the 1920s the Italian doctors, Gatti and Cayola, reported the oil to be an aphrodisiac, although no details or sources of reference were given.

One girl told me that, having decided to test the aphrodisiac properties of ylang-ylang, she gave her boyfriend a back massage with a dilution of the oil. All she would tell me was that the results were definitely out of the ordinary, since she quite often gave him a back massage. Another told me that she put a few drops of the oil in her boyfriend's bath, and later went into the bathroom. She emerged, rather wet, some two hours later, but again was reluctant to explain any further. An aromatherapist who trained with me had an interesting experience when using ylang-ylang oil on the treatment of a man who was complaining of impotence. At the time (1986) he was thirty-one years old, and had been a singer in a new-wave band, on the road for several years. He told the therapist that he had had his share of brief affairs, although he was married. One year before coming for treatment he split up with his wife and went into producing, as he could no longer handle the strain of being on the road. Since that time he had been quite impotent, and in fact had lost all desire for sex. (Impotence is quite common for a short period following a split or divorce.) The therapist used a dilution of ylang-ylang oil and jasmine, but the treatment was a little more successful than she had anticipated. The patient expressed how good he was feeling and made advances towards the therapist, who was fortunately able to handle the situation. I must emphasize that aphrodisiac oils usually only work as such when you want them to, and this situation would surely not have occurred had the therapist been male. Ylang-ylang is frequently used in aromatherapy with no *immediate* sexually stimulating result.

Another anecdote comes from Gordon Haddock:

Whilst in France last year (1986) I stayed over at a friend's villa in Cannes for a couple of weeks. During my stay I became acquainted with some people who invited me to a party. I had to be there at a certain time to get into the building, as it had quite formidable security. Having missed my rendezvous . . . I decided to scale the gates and hence make my entrance, which I did. Unfortunately an Alsatian guard dog had anticipated my arrival, and leaped out at me obviously with his mind set on attack. He unfurled his lips but, to my surprise, he did not go for the jugular, and proceeded to lick me. This became somewhat embarrassing for the security guard, who was urging the dog to do something slightly more violent, and I left the two of them engrossed in a one-way argument.

I put my good fortune down to ylang-ylang oil which I had earlier used in my bath. I have found from experience that this oil appears to generate a certain interest in me from two sources – ladies and dogs. I definitely find that it has an alluring and aphrodisiac effect on the former and a calming effect on the latter.

Others have noticed the effect which ylang-ylang has on dogs (clary sage has a similar effect). It makes dogs act in a friendly manner, and is obviously attractive. However, there are no guarantees that it is going to have such an effect on all guard dogs, and I would not advise anyone to place their complete faith in such an effect.

CHAPTER EIGHT

HOME REMEDIES

I feel ashamed asking but could you please send me a small sample of your aromatic oil. My name is Leigh and I care about people's health and I would like to be a doctor when I grow up.
Thank you,
Leigh
ps. I am 10.

(This is the complete, unexpurgated draft of a letter which I received in 1976.)

This is not primarily a how-to-treat-yourself-with-aroma-therapy book, and there is certainly not enough space in this one chapter to cover the whole subject. There are many conditions, especially the chronic ones, which can only be effectively tackled by a professional physician or therapist. However, there are also many common, relatively minor problems which can be greatly relieved or even cured, with the simple application of essential oils coupled with some common-sense advice. There is no danger here at all, so long as the guidelines laid down are followed. However, if the recipe for treating cold sores says 'fifteen drops of essential oil in 50 ml of vegetable oil' and you use fifty drops in 15 ml you are going to make your cold sores worse instead of better. The amounts and dilutions should be carefully followed.

If you have any condition which persists, or steadily worsens, *do consult a practitioner*, even if it only seems a minor problem. Small symptoms occasionally hide big problems, and often precede them. Any chronic, long-standing condition is going to need expert attention. You can certainly help, but do not try to tackle it on your own. There is a world of difference between treating yourself for an insect bite, occasional indigestion or aching muscles and trying to treat conditions like chronic bronchitis, genital herpes or kidney stones. There are a few exceptions, like rheumatism, which is basically a chronic condition. However, it is extremely common, and there is a simple and safe way of *relieving* the condition with essential oils applied externally.

The remedies and advice given in this chapter should be seen rather as first aid (for insect bites, etc.) plus stop-gap relief for certain common ailments such as period pains and insomnia. The remedies should be used occasionally rather than regularly, and remember that they will not always work for everybody.

The different ways of using essential oils

Essential oils are usually diluted before use, as they are very concentrated in their pure form. The average essential oil is seventy times more concentrated than it was in the plant it came from. Formulas follow for massage oils, inhalations, compresses, bath oils and creams.

Massage Oils

Whether for use on the face or body, the way to make up your massage oil is exactly the same. You need a completely clean, empty bottle, probably about 50 ml capacity for a body oil and a 25 ml capacity for a facial oil. All chemists stock empty bottles, and most are happy to sell you a few. If you have an empty bottle and are not sure of its capacity try looking on the bottom – the capacity in mls is usually imprinted into the glass.

When you have your bottle, let us say a 50 ml one, you will put twenty-five drops of essential oil into it. Whether you use one oil or several, the total number of drops will be the same. If you have a 25 ml bottle, you will need twelve or thirteen drops, because the number of drops you use is always half the capacity of the bottle in mls. After the essential oil, you simply top up with a good quality vegetable oil. You do not need to measure this, the bottle does that for you. The best vegetable oils are sweet almond, peach kernel and apricot kernel. Almost as good are grape seed, sunflower seed and safflower seed. When you have poured both essential and vegetable oils into your bottle, shake it, not too hard, until the oils completely mix together, and then label it. Oils made like this will keep for up to three months.

A NIGHT OIL FOR THE FACE
Suitable for any skin type, except sensitive:

geranium	1
lavender	5
sandalwood	4
ylang-ylang	2
	12 drops

Mix into 25 mls of vegetable oil, and massage sparingly into clean, dry skin before retiring. Use gentle, upward movements. As you sleep the oils gradually seep into your skin, and get to work reducing oiliness, counteracting dryness and stimulating cell renewal.

A RELAXING BODY OIL

bergamot	12
geranium	4
sandalwood	9
	———
	25 drops

Mix into 50 mls of vegetable oil. Use whenever you need to relax, or to relax someone else. It will help you to reduce tension, anxiety, insomnia, night-before nerves and so on. Massage the neck and shoulders, the abdomen, the back or the whole body. You can use this sparingly as a body rub after a bath or shower, but give your skin a chance to cool down first. It will leave you both relaxed and faintly fragrant.

AN OIL FOR ACHES AND PAINS

rosemary	10
lemongrass	6
juniper	9
	———
	25 drops

Dilute in 50 mls of vegetable oil. Use for muscular aches and pains, sprained or arthritic joints, and before or after sport or exercise.

Inhalations

These are very easy to do. You need a large bowl (the bigger the better) filled with almost boiling water. Add a total of 8–10 drops of essential oil and inhale deeply for ten minutes, leaning over the bowl. The traditional towel over the head is just to direct the steam and is an optional extra.

eucalyptus	2
lavender	2
lemon	2
tea-tree	2
	———
	8 drops
	———

Use as directed two or three times a day. This will help relieve sinus congestion, and will give some relief in coughs, colds, flu and sore throats.

An antiseptic cream

Buy a 30 g pot of unscented cream base from your local chemist, preferably one which does not contain lanolin. Add to it the following essential oils:

lavender	9
tea-tree	6
	———
	15 drops
	———

Stir the essential oils into the cream using a small, clean implement. Usually they will not separate out again. However, if they do after a few days, just stir them back in again before using the cream. You can use this for any kind of skin problem where there is infection or a risk of infection, including spots, sores, cold sores, and minor cuts and abrasions. It will also help some cases of eczema, although this really requires holistic treatment. For athlete's foot or ringworm, you will need a stronger concentration of essential oil: eighteen drops of lavender and twelve of tea-tree in the same amount of cream.

Undiluted lavender oil

Use lavender oil neat on minor burns and scalds and on insect bites and stings. Apply it every minute or two until the pain is almost gone, and then a few more times every fifteen minutes. Only a little oil is required, applied directly to the affected area. You can also use tea-tree oil in the same way, or a mixture of lavender and tea-tree.

Baths

For maximum therapeutic effect, floating oils are best, and the simplest thing to do is to use pure essential oils. After running your bath add between three and six drops of essential oil to the water. Before you get in, agitate the water so that the oils spread evenly over the surface. This means that your body picks up a very thin, even layer of oil as you enter the water and it guards against a whole drop of oil settling on your skin, which can be slightly irritating. If you have moderately sensitive skin use less, rather than more, essential oil. Now lie back, relax and enjoy. A tiny amount of essence is absorbed through the skin, but the main effect is through inhalation of the vapours. As your nose gets used to the fragrance you may not notice it after a while. Do not worry, the oils are still having an effect on your olfactory nerves and limbic system, even if the conscious mind no longer registers the odour.

A EUPHORIC BATH OIL

clary sage	2
ylang-ylang	2
	———
	4 drops

Use when you are feeling down or depressed, or when you just want to float.

A REFRESHING BATH OIL

geranium	1
orange	2
rosewood	3
	———
	6 drops
	———

Use to wake you up in the morning, and to refresh you after a hard day's work, or before an evening out.

Compresses

To make an aromatic compress you need a shallow bowl, about 25 cm in diameter. You could make do with a clean wash-hand basin. Fill the bowl with water at a temperature which feels pleasantly warm to the touch and add only one or two drops of essential oil. Agitate the water gently, so that the oils spread evenly over the surface, and then dip on to the *surface* of the water a folded handkerchief or something similar. Do not immerse it into the water. This way the handkerchief picks up a thin, even film of water and essential oil on one surface. Lay this same surface on to the skin and cover with something dry, like a small towel or scarf. Leave on for anything between fifteen minutes and an hour.

COMPRESS FOR A HANGOVER

fennel	1
juniper	1
	———
	2 drops
	———

Apply to the forehead and temples, and also over the liver, which means over the lower part of the front ribs on the right side of the body. It is also a good idea to drink lots of water.

COMPRESS FOR PERIOD PAINS

clary sage	1
cypress	1
	———
	2 drops
	———

Place over the lower abdomen, and you could also put another over the lower back.

If you do not mind, and if you can stop it from slipping, there is no reason why you should not walk around with a compress secreted under your clothes. If it feels comfortable, you can leave it on for several hours.

A Word of Warning

I have made an extensive study of the safety aspect of aromatherapy, resulting in *The Essential Oil Safety Data Manual* for therapists and researchers. Essential oils have been thoroughly tested for toxicity and irritation, since they are so widely used in the fragrance and flavour industries. Most of the hazardous oils, which include, for instance, oils of mustard, wormseed, calamus and pennyroyal, are not generally available. However, at the time of writing a few suspect oils, notably sage and thyme, have not yet been withdrawn from general use in aromatherapy.

There is no reason to believe that taking oils by mouth is more hazardous than putting them on your skin *if only a few doses are taken*. It is much more important to avoid the hazardous essential oils than it is to avoid oral ingestion, which is rapidly becoming unfashionable among UK aromatherapists. The same amount of essential oil finds its way into the bloodstream from an aromatherapy massage as from one oral dose. However, since massage is done once a week, and oral ingestion three times a day, I would not recommend anyone to take essential oils for more than a week at a time. To play safe, it would be advisable not to take essential oils orally, or to use them in any way on children of five years or under, unless under the guidance of a doctor, herbalist or aromatherapist.

Here are some safety guidelines for using essential oils at home:

These oils are not safe for home use:

origanum	thyme
sage	wintergreen
savory	

In pregnancy, avoid the above mentioned oils, plus the following:

basil	marjoram
clove	myrrh
hyssop	

These oils should not be used on the skin at all:

cinnamon   clove

These oils may cause very slight irritation on sensitive skins, especially if used in compresses or baths:

basil   rosemary
fennel   verbena
lemongrass

If you have extremely sensitive skin you may find that many, even all, essential oils are minor irritants, in which case you will have to avoid them.

The following oils should not be applied to the skin prior to sunbathing, or going under a sun-bed:

bergamot   orange
lemon   any other citrus oil
grapefruit verbena

Overall, it is best to stick to published recipes and formulas most of the time, although I cannot be responsible for those published in aromatherapy books in which I have not been involved. Please do not be put off by these few words of warning; it is not quite as bad as it sounds, but we have to be super-safe. Even the most toxic essential oils are not harmful if only one or two small doses are taken, and they are less toxic than some chemical drugs. If the safety guidelines are followed, and they are really quite simple, there is no possibility of harm being done.

USEFUL ADDRESSES

To order Essential Oils Incense or other aromatic products, please contact:

WHOLESALE	RETAIL
Lotus Light	Lotus Fulfillment Services
P.O. Box 2	33719 116th St.
Wilmot, WI 53192	Twin Lakes, WI 53181
(414) 862-2395	

Aromatherapy associations

For a list of recommended practitioners, write:

The Association of Tisserand Aromatherapists
(ATA), P.O. Box 746, Brighton BN1 3BN
The International Federation of Aromatherapists,
46 Dalkeith Road, London SE21, 8LS (England)

Aromatherapy seminars and courses

If you interested in training as an aromatherapist, write to Robert Tisserand at the ATA address above.

Robert Tisserand runs one- and two-day seminars for those who do not wish to train in aromatherapy professionally but who would like guidance in practicing it at home.

If you would like information regarding seminars or are interested in sponsoring Robert Tisserand for programs, please contact Lotus Light at the above address.

REFERENCES

1 Aromatherapy Today

1. Editorial, *Journal of Alternative Medicine*, July 1984, p. 1.
2. 'Male Chauvinism in Toxicity Testing?', *Manufacturing Chemist*, July 1983, p. 3.
3. A. Guild, 'Olfactory Acuity in Normal and Obese Subjects', *Journal of Laryngology*, vol. 70, 1956, pp. 408–14.
4. H. S. Koelega, 'Extraversion, Sex, Arousal, and Olfactory Sensitivity', *Acta Psychologica*, vol. 34, 1970, pp. 51–66.
5. C. Van Toller, G. H. Dodd, and A. Billing, *Ageing and the Sense of Smell*, Springfield, MA, 1985.

2 Nothing New

1. P. Rovesti, *In Search of Perfumes Lost*, Venice, 1980, p. 22.
2. R. Noorbergen, *Secrets of the Lost Races*, London, 1978.
3. B. Ebbell, *The Papyrus Ebers*, London, 1937.
4. C. J. Thompson, *The Mystery and Lure of Perfume*, London, 1927.
5. R. Genders, *A History of Scent*, London, 1972.
6. E. Rimmel, *The Book of Perfumes*, London, 1865.
7. R. T. Gunther, *The Greek Herbal of Dioscorides* (Translated by John Goodyer in 1655), New York, 1959.
8. G. E. R. Lloyd, *Hippocratic Writings*, London, 1978, p. 224.
9. *The Yellow Emperor's Classic of Internal Medicine*, translated by Ilza Veith, Los Angeles, 1973, p. 211.
10. R. J. Forbes, *A Short History of the Art of Distillation*, Leiden, 1970.
11. O. C. Gruner, *A Treatise on the Canon of Medicine of Avicenna*, New York, 1979, p. 390.
12. E. S. Rohde, *The Old English Herbals*, London, 1972, p. 3.
13. R. Tisserand, *The Art of Aromatherapy*, London, 1977.
14. H. Braunschweig, *New Vollkomen Distillierbuch*, Frankfurt, 1597.
15. W. H. Ryff, *Neu Gross Destillierbuch*, Frankfurt, 1545.

16. A. Lonicer, *Kräuterbuch*, Frankfurt, 1550.

17. C. Gesner, *The Treasure of Euonymus*, Zurich, 1559.

18. T. E. Knyght, *The Castel of Helth*, London, 1541.

19. L. Shih-Chen, *Chinese Medicinal Herbs* (translation of the *Pen Ts'ao*, first published in 1578), San Francisco, 1973.

20. N. Culpeper, *The English Physitian*, London, 1653.

21. J. Pechey, *The Compleat Herbal of Physical Plants*, London, 1694.

22. C. J. Thompson, *Alchemy*, London, 1897.

23. W. Whitla, *Elements of Pharmacy, Materia Medica and Therapeutics*, London, 1882.

24. Chamberland, *Annales de l'Institut Pasteur*, vol. 1, 1887, p. 153.

25. W. Minchin, 'The Germicidal and Therapeutic Action of Garlic', *Practitioner*, vol. 20, 1918, p. 145; ibid., vol. 21, 1918, pp. 145–54.

26. R. M. Gattefossé, *Aromathérapie*, Paris, 1937.

27. A. Couvreur, *Les Produits Aromatiques Utilisées en Pharmacie*, Paris, 1939.

28. J. Valnet, *The Practice of Aromatherapy*, Saffron Walden, 1980.

29. M. Maury, *Le Capital 'Jeunesse'*, Paris, 1961.

3 How It Works

1. D. L. J. Opdyke, 'Inhibition of Sensitization Reactions Induced by Certain Aldehydes', *Food and Cosmetics Toxicology*, vol. 14 (3), 1976, pp. 197–8.

2. R. Tisserand, *The Art of Aromatherapy*, London, 1977, p. 146.

3. J. Valnet, *The Practice of Aromatherapy*, Saffron Walden, 1980, p. 23.

4. L. L. Gershbein, 'Regeneration of Rat Liver in the Presence of Essential Oils and their Components', *Food and Cosmetics Toxicology*, vol. 15, 1977, pp. 173–81.

5. P. Rovesti, *In Search of Perfumes Lost*, Venice, 1980, p. 131.

6. D. Krieger, *The Therapeutic Touch: How to Use Your Hands to Help or to Heal*, Englewood Cliffs, NJ, 1982.

7. A. Montagu, *Touching: The Human Significance of the Skin*, New York, 1971.

8. F. S. Hammett, 'Studies of the Thyroid Apparatus: 1', *American Journal of Physiology*, vol. 56, 1921, pp. 196–204.

9. C. M. Kuhn et al., 'Loss of Tissue Sensitivity to Growth Hormone During Maternal Deprivation in Rats', *Life Sciences*, vol. 25, 1979, pp. 2089–97.

10. S. M. Schanberg *et al.*, 'Tactile and Nutritional Aspects of Maternal Care', *Proceedings of the Society for Experimental Biology and Medicine*, vol. 175, 1984, pp. 135–46.

11. T. Kaptchuk and M. Croucher, *The Healing Arts*, London, 1986.

12. S. Jourard, *The Transparent Self*, New York, 1971.

13. S. Sims, 'Slow Stroke Back Massage for Cancer Patients', *Nursing Times*, vol. 82 (13), 1986, pp. 47–50.

14. L. Chaitow, 'The Application of Neurological Reflexes to the Treatment of Hypertension', *Journal of the American Osteopathic Association*, vol. 79 (4), 1979, pp. 225–30.

15. C. Houseman, 'Make the Most of Yourself in 1987', *Disability Now*, January 1987, pp. 8–9.

16. D. Macht, 'The Absorption of Drugs and Poisons through the Skin and Mucous Membranes', *Journal of the American Medical Association*, vol. 110, 1938, pp. 409–14.

17. Von Fr. Meyer, and E. Meyer, 'Percutane Resorption von Ätherischen Ölen und ihren Inhaltsstoffen', *Arzneimittel-Forschung*, vol. 9, 1959, pp. 516–19.

18. P. Weintraub, 'Scentimental Journeys', *Omni*, vol. 8 (7), 1986, pp. 48–52, 114–16.

19. L. Chaitow, *Neuro-Muscular Technique*, Wellingborough, 1980, p. 39.

20. P. G. F. Nixon, 'Therapeutic Balance', private paper.

21. J. Valnet, C. Duraffourd and J. Lapraz, *Une Médecine Nouvelle*, Paris, 1978.

22. F. Caujolle *et al.*, 'Pharmacodynamic Action of Essential Oil of Hyssop', *Comptes Rendus Société Biologique*, vol. 139, 1945, p. 1111.

23. J. C. Maruzella and P. A. Henry, 'The *in vitro* Antibacterial Activity of Essential Oils and Oil Combinations', *Journal of the American Pharmaceutical Association*, vol. 47, 1958, pp. 294–6.

24. A. Kar and S. R. Jain, 'Antibacterial Evaluation of Some Indigenous Medicinal Volatile Oils', *Qual. Plant. Mater. Veg.*, vol. 20 (3), 1971, pp. 231–7.

25. J. Kabara, 'Aroma Preservatives: Essential Oils and Fragrances as Anti-Microbial Agents', *Cosmetic Science*, vol. 1, 1984, pp. 237–73.

26. Preservative Effectiveness Test (Australia), U S P 19, 1975.

27. K. Okazaki *et al.*, *J. Pharm, Soc. Japan*, vol. 73 (4), 1953, pp. 344–7.

28. S. Vichkanova *et al.*, 'Antiviral Activity Displayed by the Essential Oil of *Eucalyptus Viminalis* & Some Other Frost-Hardy Eucalypti', *Farmakol. Toxicol.* (Moscow), vol. 36 (3), 1973, pp. 339–41.

29. S. G. Ong, 'Treatment of Influenza with Volatile Oils Extracted from Chinese Plants II', *Science Record*, new ser. vol. 2 (7), 1958, pp. 233–8; also 'III', ibid., vol. 3 (3), 1959, pp. 120–27.

30. M. A. Weiner, *Maximum Immunity*, Bath, 1986.

31. R. Kobert, *Pharmakotherapie v. Ätherischen Öle*, 1906.

32. T. Okanishi, 'Some Pharmacological Action of Oils of Sandal, Pine, and Vetiver', *Fol. Pharmacol. Japon.*, vol. 7, 1928, pp. 77–85.

33. H. M. Gattefossé, article in *Perfumery and Essential Oil Record*, December 1954, pp. 406–9.

34. R. Tisserand, *The Essential Oil Safety Data Manual*, Brighton, 1985.

35. M. K. Jain and R. Apitz-Castro, 'Garlic: Molecular Basis of the Putative "Vampire-repellant" Action and Other Matters Related to Heart and Blood', *T.I.B.S.*, vol. 12, 1987, pp. 252–4.

36. I. Janku *et al.*, 'The Diuretic Principle of *Juniperus communis*', *Arch. Exptl. Pathol. Pharmakol.*, vol. 238, 1960, pp. 112–13.

5 The Psyche

1. D. Hines, 'Olfaction and the Right Cerebral Hemisphere', *Journal of Altered States of Consciousness*, vol. 3 (1), 1977, pp. 47–59.

2. P. Weintraub, 'Scentimental Journeys', *Omni*, vol. 8 (7), 1986, pp. 48–52, 114–16.

3. C. Clifford, 'New Scent Waves', *Self*, December 1985, pp. 115–17.

4. S. Schiffman, 'Multidimensional Analysis of Odours', *Science*, vol. 185, 1974, pp. 112–16.

5. A. Baumeister, 'Suppression of Repetitive Self-injurious Behaviour by Contingent Inhalation of Aromatic Ammonia', *Journal of Autism and Childhood Schizophrenia*, vol. 8, 1978, pp. 71–7.

6. M. D. Kirk-Smith, C. Van Toller and G. H. Dodd, 'Unconscious Odour Conditioning in Human Subjects', *Biological Psychology*, vol. 17, 1983, pp. 221–3.

7. T. Engen *et al.*, 'Long-term Memory of Odours with and without Verbal Descriptors', *Journal of Experimental Psychology*, vol. 100, 1973, pp. 221–7.

8. L. Bolloré, 'Special Parfum', *Vogue*, no. 671, November, 1986, p. 288.

9. G. J. Tortora and N. P. Anagnostakos, *Principles of Anatomy and Physiology*, New York, 1984.

10. C. Van Toller, 'Emotion, and Brain Imaging of Reactions to Smells', in *Perfumery: The Psychology and Biology of Fragrance*, London, 1988.

11. J. Valnet, *The Practice of Aromatherapy*, Saffron Walden, 1980.

12. H. Gordon *et al.*, 'Lateralisation of Olfactory Perception in the Surgically Separated Hemispheres of Man', *Neuropsychologia*, vol. 7, 1969, pp. 111–20.

13. C. Van Toller *et al.*, 'Skin Conductance and Subjective Assessments Associated with the Odour of Androstanone', *Biological Psychology*, vol. 16, 1983, pp. 85–107.

14. P. Rovesti *et al.*, 'Aromatherapy and Aerosols', *Soap, Perfumery and Cosmetics*, vol. 46 (8), 1973, pp. 475–7.

15. G. Gatti and R. Cayola, 'L'Azione delle essenze sul sistema nervoso', *Rivista Italiana Essenze e Profumi*, vol. 5 (12), 1923, pp. 133–5.

16. P. Rovesti, *In Search of Perfumes Lost*, Venice, 1980.

17. R. Tisserand, 'Essential Oils as Psychotherapeutic Agents', in *Perfumery: The Psychology and Biology of Fragrance*, London, 1988.

18. D. I. Macht *et al.*, 'Sedative Properties of Some Aromatic Drugs and Fumes', *Journal of Pharmacology*, vol. 18 (5), 1921, pp. 361–72.

19. S. Torii *et al.*, 'Measuring the Mood of a Fragrance', in *Perfumery: The Psychology and Biology of Fragrance*, London, 1988.

7 Essential Oils

1. F. Cola, *Le Livre du Parfumeur*, Paris, 1931.

2. R. Tisserand, *The Art of Aromatherapy*, London, 1977.

3. S. Atanassova-Shopova and K. Roussinov, 'Effects of *Salvia sclarea* Essential Oil on the Central Nervous System', *Bulletin of the Institute of Physiology, Bulgarian Academy of Sciences*, vol. 13, 1970, pp. 89–95.

4. J. Valnet, *The Practice of Aromatherapy*, Saffron Walden, 1980, p. 23.

5. R. M. Gattefossé, 'L'Aromathérapie en Amerique', *La Parfumerie Moderne*, 1935, pp. 409–11.

6. 'All in a Doctor's Day', *Sunday Express*, 18 November, 1979.

7. L. Shih-Chen, *Chinese Medicinal Herbs* (translation of the *Pen Ts'ao*, first published in 1578, San Francisco, 1973, p. 381.

8. E. Vasileva *et al.*, 'Choleretic Action of Rose Oil in Tests on Rats', *Farmakol. Toxicol.* (Moscow), vol. 35 (3), 1972, pp. 312–15.

9. A. Maleev *et al.*, Bulgarian Rose Oil: Pharmacological and Clinical Investigations. (Rosanol) 1974.

10. E. Humphery, 'A New Australian Germicide', *Medical Journal of Australia*, January 1930, p. 417.

11. A. Penfold, 'Some Notes on the Essential Oil of *Melaleuca alternifolia*', *Australian Journal of Pharmocology*, March 1937, p. 274.

12. M. Walker, 'Clinical Investigation of Australian *Melaleuca alternifolia* Oil for a Variety of Common Foot Problems', *Current Podiatry*, April 1972.

13. E. Peña, '*Melaleuca alternifolia* Oil: its Use for Trichomonal Vaginitis and Other Vaginal Infections', *Obstetrics and Gynecology*, vol. 19 (6), 1962, pp. 793–5.

14. P. Belaiche, 'Treatment of Vaginal Infections of *Candida albicans* with the Essential Oil of *Melaleuca alternifolia*', *Phytothérapie*, vol. 15, 1985, pp. 13–15.

15. P. Belaiche, 'Germicidal Properties of the Essential Oil of *Melaleuca alternifolia* Related to Urinary Infections and Chronic Ideopathic Colibaccillus', *Phytothérapie*, vol. 15, 1985, pp. 9–11.

16. Preservative Effectiveness Test (Australia), USP 19, 1975.

FURTHER READING

Kaptchuk, T., and Croucher, M., *The Healing Arts*, BBC Publications, London, 1986

Krieger, D., *The Therapeutic Touch: How to Use Your Hands to Help or to Heal*, Prentice-Hall, Englewood Cliffs, NJ, 1982

Montagu, A., *Touching: The Human Significance of the Skin*, Harper & Row, New York, 1971

Tisserand, M., *Aromatherapy for Women*, Thorsons, Wellingborough, 1985

Tisserand, R., *The Art of Aromatherapy*, C. W. Daniels, Saffron Walden, 1977

Valnet, J., *The Practice of Aromatherapy*, C. W. Daniels, Saffron Walden, 1980

Van Toller, S. and Dodd, G. H. (eds), *Perfumery: The Psychology and Biology of Fragrance*, Chapman & Hall, London, 1988

Weiner, M., *Maximum Immunity*, Gateway Books, Bath, Avon, 1986

INDEX

AYURVEDA: The Science of Self-Healing

Dr. Vasant Lad

$9.95; 176 pp;
5½ × 8½; paper
ISBN: 0-914955-00-4

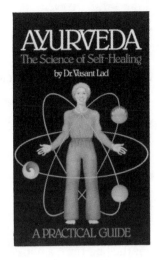

For the first time a book is available which clearly explains the principles and practical applications of Ayurveda, the oldest healing system in the world. The beautifully illustrated text thoroughly explains the following:

History & Philosophy • Basic Principles
Diagnostic Techniques • Treatment • Diet
Medical Usage of Kitchen Herbs & Spices
First Aid • Food Antidotes • And much more

More than 50 concise charts, diagrams, tables, many photographs and a full glossary and index complete this most helpful guide.

THE YOGA OF HERBS

An Ayurvedic Guide to Herbal Medicine

Dr. David Frawley and
Dr. Vasant Lad

$13.70 Postpaid
ISBN: 0941-524248

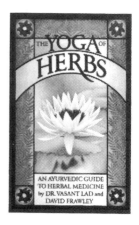

For the first time, a book is available which offers a detailed understanding and classification of herbs, utilizing the ancient system of Ayurveda. This fully developed and theoretically articulated medical system developed in India has proved itself effective for more than 5000 years as that country's classical healing tradition.

There are more than 230 herbs listed, with 88 herbs explained in detail. Included are nearly all the most commonly used western herbs according to a new and profound Ayurvedic perspective. Also a number of special powerful Ayurvedic herbs are introduced for the first time. The book is over 250 pages, with beautiful diagrams and lengthy charts, as well as a detailed glossary and index to further enhance and clarify the text.

The book combines the knowledge and experience of two respected authors in the realm of the spiritual and medical sciences of India.

Contents include:
- The Ayurvedic Theory of Herbal Medicine
- How to Prepare and Use Herbs According to Ayurveda
- Spiritual Usages of Herbs
- How to Use Herbs According to Individual Constitutional Needs
- How to Approach Western Herbs According to Ayurvedic Medical Principles

— A Y U R V E D A —

Since before 3000 B.C., Ayurveda has been the natural healing science of India, now making major inroads in the West today; in the forefront of self-care for body, mind and spirit.

HERBAL ENERGETICS CHART, edited by David Frawley, is adapted from *The Yoga of Herbs*, co-authored by David Frawley and Dr. Vasant Lad. This book's impact has already been experienced in the world of western herbology. For the first time western herbs have been systematically placed in an energetic classification, according to Ayurveda. In addition, the best selling introductory text in the field of Ayurveda entitled, *Ayurveda, The Science of Self-Healing*, authored by Dr. Vasant Lad, and *The Yoga of Herbs*, together, have sold more than 50,000 copies to date.

This chart offers practical information on 50 common western herbs, and several important Indian herbs, including:
- part of herb used
- taste
- energy
- elements
- therapeutics
- conditions
- preparation

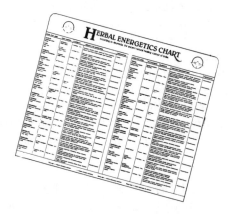

In addition, there is an explanation of Ayurveda, and a glossary describing unfamiliar terms. This simple, beautifully designed, colored laminated chart is practical and easy to use—a must for anyone interested in herbs.

$4.95; 10½ x 13½; ISBN: 0941524-29-9

PUBLISHED BY LOTUS PRESS

PLANETARY HERBOLOGY

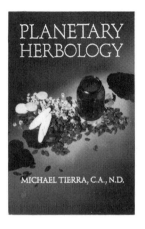

Michael Tierra, C.A., N.D.

$16.95; 485 pp.;
5½ × 8½ paper; charts.
ISBN: 0941-524272

Lotus Press is pleased to announce a new practical handbook and reference guide to the healing herbs, a landmark publication in this field. For unprecedented usefulness in practical applications, the author provides a comprehensive listing of the more than 400 medicinal herbs available in the west. They are classified according to their chemical constituents, properties and actions, indicated uses and suggested dosages. Students of eastern medical theory will find the western herbs cross-referenced to the Chinese and Ayurvedic (Indic) systems of herbal therapies. This is a useful handbook for practitioners as well as readers with a general interest in herbology.

Michael Tierra, C.A., N.D., whose very popular earlier book, *THE WAY OF HERBS,* led the way to this new major work. He is one of this country's most respected herbalists, a practitioner and teacher who has taught and lectured widely. His eclectic background studies in American Indian herbalism, the herbal system of Dr. John Christopher, and traditional oriental systems of India and China, contributes a special richness to his writing.

To order your copy, send $18.95 (postpaid) to:
LOTUS LIGHT
P.O. BOX 2
WILMOT, WI 53192